Discovering Natural Foods

For Emily.

Discovering Natural Foods

*An informative and entertaining guide
to those interesting products
in health and natural food stores*

By
Roy Bruder, Ph.D.

Foreword by
John A. Scharffenberg, M.D., M.P.H.

Illustrated by
Roni Lavine

Published by
Woodbridge Press Publishing Company
Santa Barbara, California 93111

Published and distributed by

Woodbridge Press Publishing Company
Post Office Box 6189
Santa Barbara, California 93111

Copyright © 1982 by Roy Bruder

All rights reserved.

This book or any portion thereof may not be reproduced or copied in any manner or by any means except as provided by law or as brief excerpts incorporated in a critique or review of the book, without the written permission of the publisher.

Published simultaneously in the United States and Canada.

Printed in the United States of America.

Library of Congress Cataloging in Publication Data

Bruder, Roy.
   Discovering natural foods.

  Bibliography p.
  Includes index.
  1. Food, Natural. I. Title.
TX369.B78   641.3'02   82-2705
ISBN 0-912800-86-0   AACR2

Contents

Preface   13

CHAPTER
1. What Are Natural Foods?   17
2. Transition   41
3. On the Fringe   45
4. The Protein Problem   53
5. Oils   67
6. Grains   87
7. Beans and Peas   105
8. Breakfast Cereals   117
9. Flour, Baked Goods, and Pasta   131
10. Sweeteners   157
11. Nuts, Seeds, and Dried Fruits   175
12. Snacks   197
13. Sprouts   203
14. Dairy Products, Eggs, and Substitutes   211
15. Condiments, Seasonings, Soups, and Seaweed   229
16. Juice and Other Drinks   237
17. Meat and Meat Substitutes   247
18. Supplementary Foods   255
19. Herbs, Spices, and Teas   263
20. Appliances   271
21. Putting It All Together   276

Notes   282
Index   287

Recipe Acknowledgments

1. Adapted from: *Tofu Goes West*, by Gary Landgrebe, Fresh Press, Palo Alto, CA 94303. Used by permission.
2. Adapted from: *The Farm Vegetarian Cookbook*, Louise Hagler (ed.), Copyright© 1979, The Book Publishing Co., Summertown, TN 38483. Used by permission.
3. Adapted from: *Laurel's Kitchen, A Handbook for Vegetarian Cookery & Nutrition;* by Laurel Robertson, Carol Flinders and Bronwen Godfrey. Copyright© 1976 by Nilgiri Press, Petaluma, CA 94953. Used by permission.
4. *Light Eating for Survival*, by Marcia Acciardo, Omangod Press, Woodstock Valley, CT 02682. Used by permission.
5. *Making the Change*, by Mary A. McDougell and John A. McDougall, M.D. McDougall, Kailua, HI 96734. Used by permission.
6. *Sweet Talk*, by John A. Scharffenberg, M.D., Concerned Communications, Arroyo Grande, CA 93420. Used by permission.
7. *The Oats, Peas, Beans & Barley Cookbook*, by Edyth Young Cottrell, Woodbridge Press, Santa Barbara CA 93111. Used by permission.
8. *The Pritikin Program for Diet and Exercise*, Copyright© 1979 by Nathan Pritikin and Patrick McGrady, Jr., Grosset and Dunlap, New York, N.Y. 10010. Used by permission.
9. *Recipes for a Small Planet*, by Ellen B. Ewald, Copyright© 1975, Ballantine Books, New York, N.Y. 10022. Used by permission.

Foreword

This book is for everyone who wants to change his life for the better. It is for those who have been into fast foods, or who have been among "the junk food junkies." It is for those who want to feed their families better; for those who have insight to see the writing on the wall suggesting the possibility of heart attack, cancer, stroke, diabetes, confinement to nursing homes, or premature death unless their eating habits are changed.

This book is the common meeting place of East and West; the meeting place of the scientist and the health food enthusiast. Written by a Ph.D. (physiological psychology), it cuts through fallacies sometimes heard in health food circles but at the same time is not derailed by spurious scientific reasoning. Natural foods become the natural meeting place of the nutritionist and those hoping for a "miracle" through special foods.

As we progress from those good things found in the older-style health food store to abundant good foods in the natural food stores; from some natural foods in co-ops to bulk supplies even in some large market chains; more people will discover that wholesome food as direct from the garden-to-table as possible is a treasure. This book demonstrates clearly the need for and value of such good food.

Discovering Natural Foods takes you through the natural foods in today's good stores and tells you what's what. Roy Bruder is one who knows, one who operated natural food stores for a number of years and one who has the disciplined background to analyze and evaluate.

As a nutritionist, I recommend this book to you as an aid in learning the facts about natural foods. Read on with enjoyment and make personal use of the ideas presented—for better health.

John A. Scharffenberg, M.D., M.P.H.
Associate Professor of Applied Nutrition
Loma Linda University

Acknowledgments

Many thanks to Dr. U. D. Register, Ph.D., Dr. Kenneth Burke, Ph.D., Dr. John McDougall, M.D., and Bob Petersen, M.P.H., for their efforts toward helping to maintain the credibility of the manuscript, and to my good friends Harold Payne and Frank Curcio for their many suggestions regarding style.

Special thanks goes to Dr. John A. Scharffenberg, M.D., M.P.H., who took many long hours out of his busy schedule to keep me on course and help me to avoid the temptations of half-science and overstatement.

Finally, thanks to my wife Jan, for her tolerance of all the hassles which inevitably accompany a project such as this, and for putting up with me in general.

None of the above mentioned individuals should be held responsible for any statements made in this book.

Some of the recipes at the end of each chapter are used by the gracious permission of publications shown.

Preface

The title of this book should probably have been *What Do You Do with All This Stuff, Anyhow?*, for it was that unrelenting question which led to its inception. During my years in the natural foods business, I have always felt hamstrung by the lack of a single, reasonably comprehensive source of information concerning the nature, value, and practical use of whole foods. People often came into our stores, obviously curious, obviously sensing there was something of importance going on there, but unable to overcome the sensory overload. Clearly, this was not your ordinary grocery store. Other shoppers were bustling about scooping up bags of this or that weird looking thing, appearing to know exactly what they were doing—black beans, brown rice, wheat berries, alfalfa sprouts, carob powder—and is that really green spaghetti I see over there?

Some of these newcomers wandered out as fast as they wandered in, shaking their heads and mumbling, further convinced that the world had gone mad; others remained, slack-jawed, practicing their best befuddled looks. After the culture shock had settled in a bit, I usually strolled over and put them immediately at ease by saying something like, "Why do I get the feeling this is your first time in a natural food store?" At this crucial point they either (a) ran out the door, or (b) popped the question—"What do you do with all this stuff, anyhow?"

They are asking, of course, for the impossible—a personal guided tour of the world of natural foods, a course in nutrition, and a cooking class—all in three and a half minutes. What would be nice, I thought, is if you could give them a few minutes in the way of succinct introduction and then put a book in their hands and say, "If you're really interested in learning about all this, this should tell you almost everything you'll need to get started." I am hoping that this is that book.

A perfectly reasonable question that might be asked here is: Why should you trust me? Why should you believe what I say when it often clearly contradicts what you have heard others say? Health food stores are overflowing with books, some well-intentioned, some self-serving; all expressing conflicting points of view. With a few notable exceptions, I have found these books to be largely exercises in First Amendment rights, which allow authors to say whatever they want regardless of whether or not it's true. Anecdotes are offered as "evidence," and opinion is represented as "fact" or at least not identified as opinion. Just because someone's grandmother experienced miraculous relief from her arthritis after eating such-and-such does not constitute a scientific truth. Careful observations of substantial numbers of people are necessary before inferences can be drawn, and well-designed, controlled experimentation is required before facts may be proclaimed.

I have tried my best to stay as close to the known facts as possible without becoming so rigid as to make any practical recommendations impossible. Those few authors who have elected to stay close to the facts will, for the most part, agree with what I have put forth here. And this is to be expected, since we are drawing from roughly the same body of evidence. Only our interpretations or emphases may differ.

The approach is decidedly pragmatic. It is of limited value for the newcomer to know that this grain or that bean was introduced to the North American continent by early Dutch settlers or passed along by nomadic Indian tribes. It will still taste lousy if you don't prepare it properly.

Essentially, I have tried to answer three very broad but central questions: (1) What are natural foods? (2) Why should I eat them? and (3) How do I select, store, and prepare them? Hopefully, in answering these questions, I have provided enough information for the reader to see the positive value of a natural food diet and the ease of adapting to it.

Moreover, I have tried to show that the natural food diet can be rewarding not only because of its health benefits but because it simply tastes good. It is one thing to tell people what they should or should not eat if they want to live longer and more productive lives, but quite another to expect them to subsist on bland lifeless food in pursuit of that end. The old cliche that everything good is immoral, illegal, or fattening is clever but reflects an attitude rather than a reality. Food does not have to be loaded with sugar, salt, and fat to taste pleasurable. The simplest staple foods can be made into enormously satisfying meals by the creative use of sauces, spices, and herbs, and without any special culinary genius.

Every attempt was made to be fair—fair to the consumer, fair to the retailer, fair to the manufacturer. It is unfortunate that being fair to one too often conflicts with being fair to another; but whenever this was the case the consumer held precedence. We at all levels of the natural foods business have a unique obligation to purge deception and misrepresentation from our industry. Natural food is honest food, and dishonesty has no place in its manufacture or marketing.

Roy Bruder

P.S. For the record, I confess to having used the term "Man" when I meant "humans," and the pronoun "he" when I meant "he or she." This was done in the interest of creating smoothly flowing sentences and not out of any disrespect for half the world's population.

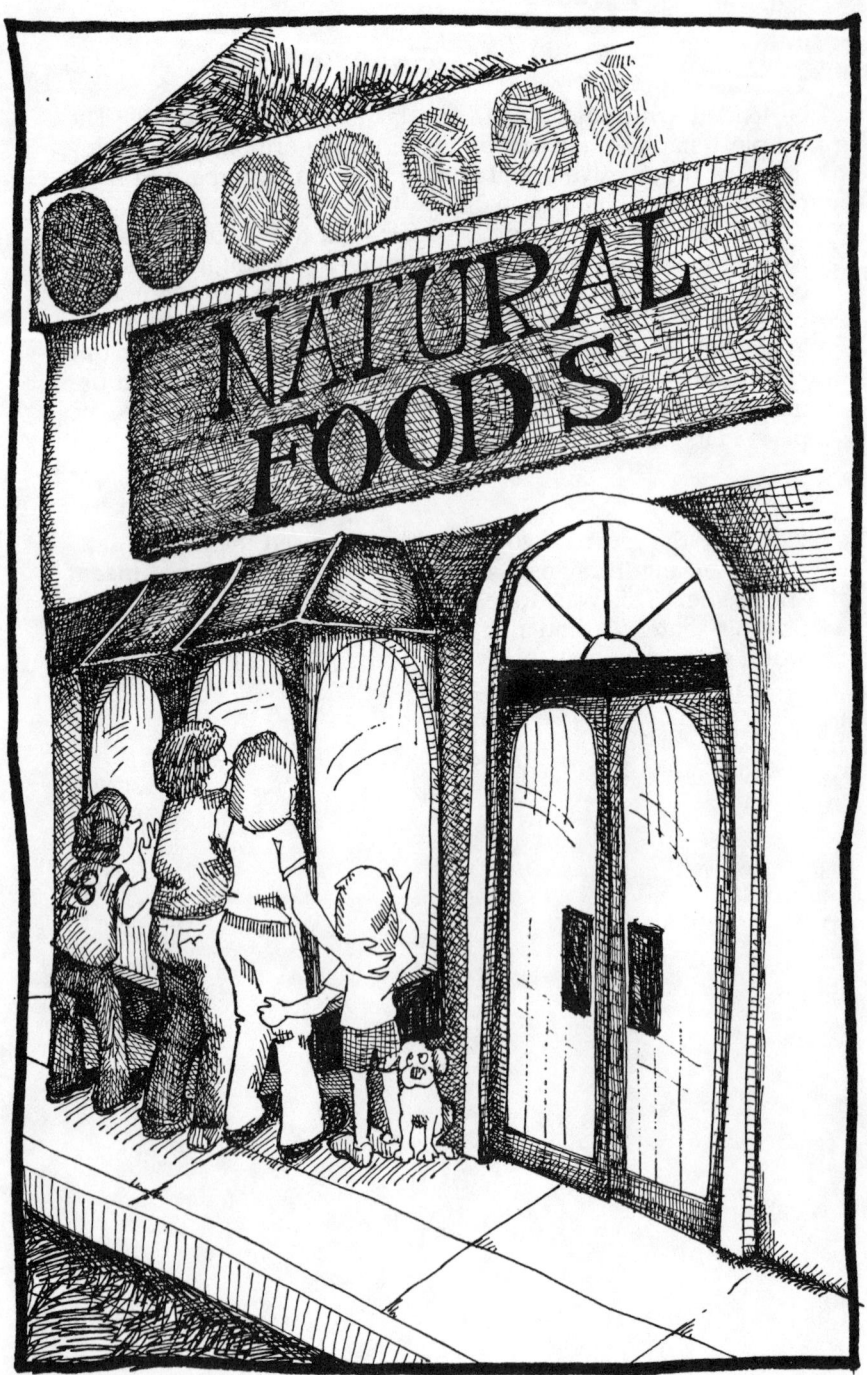

CHAPTER 1

What Are Natural Foods?

Before we talk about the pleasures of natural foods, we must set down a working definition—a guideline by which to judge the "naturalness" of any food. Let us first distinguish between the "natural food store" and the "health food store."

The term "health foods," to me, has always conjured up images of Gaylord Hauser, Adelle Davis, and gaggles of little old ladies in southern California eating wheat germ, blackstrap molasses, yeast, and God-knows-what-else for breakfast. The original health food stores were little more than glorified pharmacies; shelf after shelf of dusty little bottles of vitamin pills with a placebo for every occasion. Catering largely to senior citizens and hypochondriacs, health food stores began proliferating in the late 1950s and early 1960s particularly in California, a state which has never had any problem meeting its quota for senior citizens or hypochondriacs.

As time went on, health food stores began responding to their customers' requests for more "real food" items, and before long new shelves were added for all manner of health cookies, candies, cereals, and so forth. These products were mostly manufactured by the same people who stocked the supermarket shelves—substitute whole wheat flour for white, honey for sugar, leave out a few chemicals, jack up the price, and call it health food. Free enterprise in action.

It is difficult to say where the transition really started. Perhaps it was the change in consciousness among young people brought about by Woodstock, Vietnam, anti-establishment protest, and no doubt the ecology movement. But somewhere along the line people started to be more concerned about their bodies and what they put into them. Several classic books, like Rachel Carson's *Silent Spring*, which exposed the horrors of DDT, and Adelle Davis's *Let's Eat Right to Keep Fit*, although fraught with inaccuracies, started millions of people thinking that perhaps we are, in fact, what we eat.

People now wanted more and more to get back to basics and back to nature. They wanted to breathe clean air, drink unpolluted water, and most of all eat pure food—food that was unprocessed, unsprayed, and unchemicalized—food from the Earth rather than the laboratory.

The health food stores for the most part were unable to meet these new demands and continued to specialize in vitamin pills, which the new people viewed with the same suspicion they did Cool Whip and TV dinners.

So, in the late 1960s and early 1970s a new breed of store began to appear on the scene in places like Berkeley, San Diego, and near major college campuses throughout the U.S. They started either as co-ops, where the customers contributed a certain amount of labor in exchange for the privilege of buying food at prices only marginally above cost, or as ordinary retail proprietorships. Regardless of their particular business structure, they shared the same goal: to offer consumers a central marketplace for unrefined natural food, free of chemical additives.

The new natural food markets were alternative grocery stores—alternatives to the drugstore-like sterility of the health food store and the impersonality and deception of the giant supermarket chains, where your basic breakfast treat may contain more sugar than cereal.

In the beginning, of course, the idea that Funky Fred's Natural Foods could present any serious challenge to Safeway was laughable. Today, no one is laughing. *Natural Foods Merchandiser* reported in 1981 that health and natural food stores were capturing better than $2.4 billion from consumers annually and this figure is going nowhere but up. Major supermarkets (including Safeway) are now scrambling to stock natural food items on their shelves to meet consumer demands, and supermarket-size natural food stores are now cropping up all over the Southwest, some doing upwards of $10 million in annual sales.

Although some health food stores still avoid stocking very much in the way of real food items, and a few ultra-pure natural food stores refuse to sell vitamin supplements, most have integrated their inventories sufficiently to meet the needs of a wider variety of customers. Health food stores now routinely carry packages of brown rice, granola, whole grain breads, raw dairy products, nuts, seeds, and so forth, while many natural food stores offer token amounts of vitamins for customer convenience. But in general the distinction remains, primarily due to the emphasis placed upon whole foods versus supplements.

Another qualitative difference is the tendency of most natural food stores to offer their customers the opportunity of buying commodities "in bulk." A typical store consists of hundreds of bins filled with grains, beans, pasta, nuts, seeds, dried fruit, flour, and much more, from which the customer may scoop up and weigh out just what he needs rather than be forced to buy pre-packaged amounts. There is an obvious economic advantage to this type of buying: the expense of packaging, weighing, and elaborate labelling is eliminated.

A Definition

Nutrition is like religion—there are devoted followers of each school of thought and total agreement among them is difficult to imagine. So any definition of natural foods is implicitly arbitrary to some degree. Some would say that only a food in its whole, natural state, i.e., as grown by nature, unprocessed and unchanged in any manner, qualifies. Fruit juice, for example, falls short of so strict a definition since it is derived from natural foods but in its current form represents a "fraction," lacking the fiber present in the whole fruit. Oatmeal, or rolled oats as they are often called, also fails to qualify since the whole oat is changed from its natural form and some deterioration inevitably occurs. Pragmatically speaking, this is extremism, and in spite of the fact that these people are technically correct, in reality the overwhelming bulk of humans are not going to eat that way. A working definition must be tempered and molded to fit the culture it must serve; otherwise it is useful only to those who write textbooks. A more practical definition might look like this: a *natural food*
  1. is a whole, unprocessed food or a food derived from a whole food containing all or most of the nutrients of the original source;
  2. contains no artificial substances;

3. is a fit food for human consumption, in that its effect on the health of the body is predominantly positive.

Let's pick this apart a little and examine the criteria presented. "Whole, unprocessed foods" are those which the Earth has given us: whole fruits, vegetables, nuts, seeds, grains, beans, etc., with only the inedible parts removed. No problem here. "Derived foods" gets a little hazier. Obviously, pure unfiltered and unpasteurized apple juice is a derived food, but basically a good one since it contains most of its original nutrients. Rolled, cracked, or milled grains contain most of the nutrients present in the original food, although some are routinely destroyed simply by exposure to air. Well then, what about white flour? Is it not in fact derived from a whole food? Yes, but so many of the nutrients have been removed in processing that any resemblance to whole wheat is purely coincidental. And even if it is "enriched" white flour, to which a few synthetic nutrients have been added, it is still deficient in many key substances. Although, technically speaking, laboratory vitamins are identical to natural vitamins, they are nevertheless man-made, and so enriched white flour dosed with these man-made substances would violate our second criterion.

Part two also deals with those foods containing BHA, BHT, sodium benzoate, polysorbate 60, red dye #40, and any other of the more than 5000 chemicals used regularly to dose our daily bread. Clearly, these are not natural foods.

The final criterion will probably involve the most decision making on your part. After considering all the available information, you will be able to determine for yourself whether a food, like beef, for example, has enough nutritional benefits to outweigh the drawbacks presented by such things as its high saturated fat and cholesterol content.

We can, at this point, make a sort of laundry list of those foods commonly found in the typical American diet which do not meet our criteria for natural foods. A quick reading of the following chart will serve to introduce the concept, and each key food will be discussed in greater detail later on.

Abstracting the information from this chart, we can rephrase it in a series of statements regarding what is wrong with the typical Western diet.

1. It is too high in fat, particularly saturated fat.
2. It is too high in cholesterol.
3. It is too high in protein.

What Are Natural Foods?

Food	Criteria Violated	Reasons
animal fats (butter, lard)	1, 2, 3	—too high in saturated fat and cholesterol —a fraction of a more complete food; no fiber —may contain environmental toxins and additives
vegetable oil	1, 3, sometimes 2	—an empty calorie food with little nutritional benefit —too high in fat (100%) —oxidizes to form substances believed to be carcinogenic —may contain additives
white flour and its products	1, 2	—too refined; nutrient deficient, too low in fiber —may contain additives
white rice	1, sometimes 2	—too refined; lacking in nutrients and fiber —may be coated with asbestos talc
refined sugars: white sugar, raw sugar, honey, molasses, maple syrup, etc.	1, 3	—empty calorie foods; no benefit other than pure carbohydrate (except molasses which contains some minerals) —too refined; absorbed into system too rapidly
salt	3	—OK in small amounts, but harmful above 5 grams per day; causes high blood pressure
meat, poultry	2, 3	—contain chemical residues —too high in fat, cholesterol, protein, and salt —lacking in carbohydrate and fiber

scaly fish	3, sometimes 2	—too high in cholesterol and protein —lacking in carbohydrate and fiber —may contain environmental toxins and heavy metals
shellfish	2, 3	—too high in cholesterol, and protein —lacking in carbohydrate and fiber —are scavengers and may contain environmental toxins
milk, cheese, and all other milk products	3, sometimes 2	—too high in fat, cholesterol, and protein —lacking in carbohydrate and fiber —may contain environmental toxins and additives
eggs	3	—too high in fat, cholesterol and protein —lacking in carbohydrate and fiber
all foods containing artificial preservatives, colors, flavors, emulsifiers, stabilizers, etc.	2	—additives may be problematic

4. It is too high in refined foods, especially refined carbohydrates (sugar, white flour), and refined fats.
5. It is too high in salt.
6. It is too low in dietary fiber.
7. It is too low in complex carbohydrates.
8. It contains too many laboratory chemicals about which we know little.

Now that I have somewhat shaken your concept of diet, let me attempt to defend each of these statements with the available scientific evidence and a touch of common sense.

Fat

The typical Western diet contains 40 percent fat. That is to say, 40 percent of the total calories taken in as food on a daily basis are from fat. This is entirely too high, not only because that amount of fat is harmful, but also because the fat replaces (by adding calories) other foods which would be far more beneficial. Most responsible experts in this field suggest we reduce our fat consumption to at least half that figure, to 20 percent or even as low as 10 percent. This will obviously involve some restructuring of the diet. In addition, experts suggest we shift the emphasis of our remaining fat intake from one type of fat to another.

Fats may be divided into three general categories: *saturated*, *monounsaturated*, and *polyunsaturated*. Although most natural foods which contain fat possess all three types, it is the proportions in which they are found, rather than the absolute amount of fat, that determines their degree of desirability in the diet.

Saturated fats are the hard, solid fats found predominantly in animal products, i.e., meat, milk, cheese, butter, eggs, and so forth. Monounsaturated fats, although found in most foods containing fats, appear in abundance in only one common food, the olive. Polyunsaturated fats are the main fats found in plant foods, i.e., nuts, seeds, beans, grains, and vegetables in general. These rules are not without exception. Coconut, a plant food, is extremely high in saturated fat, the highest in fact; whereas fish is often quite low in saturated fat and high in polyunsaturates.

Of the three types of fat, saturated appears to be the most problematic, since it causes blood cholesterol levels to rise and this condition appears to be strongly associated with coronary artery disease.[1] Also, a high saturated fat diet results in the production of large amounts of bile acid, which may be a cause of colon cancer.[2]

A third problem with saturated fat is that it causes the red blood cells to clump together and line up like a stack of poker chips. This slows blood circulation and decreases oxygen uptake by vital tissues for up to nine hours.[3] Ever wonder why everyone falls asleep after Thanksgiving dinner? All that meat, fatty gravy, butter, eggs, and cream so overload the blood stream with saturated fat the brain is deprived of sufficient oxygen to carry on normal waking activities (cerebral anoxia).[4]

Polyunsaturates have been shown to be cholesterol-lowering in human and animal systems, and taken alone this information would lead us to look upon them favorably. Other evidence, unfortunately, tends to dampen our enthusiasm, since polyunsaturated oils have been associated with an increased incidence of cancer in laboratory animals in some, but not all, studies.[5]

For the record, monounsaturates neither lower nor raise cholesterol levels, and at least in this respect seem to be neutral fats.[6]

The concept of fat and oil in the diet is most important and for this reason will be discussed in greater detail in Chapters 4 and 5.

Cholesterol

Cholesterol is a substance produced only in animal systems (including ours) and found only in foods of animal origin. No vegetable food contains cholesterol. There is, however, a small hook to this. Cholesterol levels are raised in human systems either by: (a) ingesting foods high in cholesterol; or (b) ingesting foods high in saturated fat, since the presence of an abundance of saturated fat in the blood causes normal cholesterol production to increase, or at least causes the body to retain more cholesterol. So eating an avocado, for example, especially high in saturated fat, will result in elevated cholesterol levels in spite of the fact that it contains no cholesterol of its own. This is why persons on diets designed to lower blood cholesterol levels are restricted from eating avocado, although it is a perfectly good food for those with healthy cholesterol readings.

If you want to reduce your cholesterol level, obviously you must reduce your intake of foods rich in cholesterol and saturated fat. This will include all but the leanest meats, whole milk, butter, cheese, yogurt, ice cream, egg yolks, shellfish, avocado, and certain hydrogenated vegetable oils (discussed in Chapter 5).

The obvious question here is: Why should I be concerned about my cholesterol level? The answer is that although all the votes have not yet been counted, preliminary returns indicate that high cholesterol levels are strongly associated with heart disease. The lack of consensus on the importance of cholesterol among experts has resulted in general confusion on the part of the public. While some view cholesterol as a dominant health

hazard, others advise you to ignore such admonitions and eat whatever you want. Consider the following:
1. In populations where cholesterol levels are high, so is the incidence of heart disease, and vice versa.[7]
2. In individuals, this has been more difficult to show. However, there are some good specific correlations between heart attacks and certain aspects of cholesterol level.[8]
3. Those experts who claim cholesterol is harmless usually seem to be financially supported to some degree by the meat, egg, and dairy industries.

While it is true that cholesterol is an essential body substance and is naturally produced by your own system, there is no evidence that any cholesterol is needed from the diet. My feeling is that if a substance is unnecessary, if there is substantial evidence that it is harmful, and if the foods in which it occurs appear to be problematic in their own right, why take the risk? There is nothing magical about any of these cholesterol-containing foods. No nutrient which they provide cannot readily be obtained from other sources.

Protein

Our typical Western diet derives 15 percent of its calories from protein, and this is greatly in excess of what is actually required by the body. A more reasonable proportion would be 10 percent of our daily caloric intake from protein, although as low as 5 percent would be adequate.[9] Now, if excess protein were simply passed out of the body harmlessly, we shouldn't have to worry about taking in too much. Unfortunately, this is not the case. Our bodies require a certain amount of protein for general maintenance (e.g., rebuilding cells that have died natural deaths or have been destroyed by injury or illness) and has a very small capacity for storage, but excess amounts must be eliminated. These rather large molecules are excreted for the most part through the kidneys, and it's not easy work. Excess protein is passed only at great expense, and the more you eat the more you overwork these vital organs.[10]

The second problem with too much protein is the tendency to increase the urinary excretion of calcium. Too much calcium is drawn from the bones resulting in the eventual "softening" and weakening of basic structural elements.[11] When Grandma slips on the sidewalk and breaks her hip and it takes six months to heal, everyone attributes it to the curse of old age. It is, in fact, the result of a common condition known as *osteoporosis;* too much calcium has been leached from her bones. This is not an inevitable but a preventable condition. Studies have shown that protein intakes of more than 75 grams per day may not be wise.[12]

Finally, there is the problem of uric acid production. Substances common to all protein known as nucleic acids induce the formation of uric acid, the crystals of which deposit in the bone joints and produce a condition known as gout. Gout often begins with a sore toe or sore knuckles and progresses to painful swelling of many joints in the body. Gout is, for the most part, preventable.

Refined Carbohydrates

When whole wheat flour is processed into white flour, and brown rice polished into white, we have what are known as refined carbohydrates. They still possess the caloric value of the original carbohydrate, often much of the protein, and some small measure of vitamins and minerals, but they are decidedly deficient in many important nutrients and especially dietary fiber.

The main problem with refined carbohydrates is that they replace foods in the diet that would provide more nutrition for the calories gained. Nowhere is this more flagrant than in the case of refined sugars, which have few if any nutrients other than pure carbohydrate. Refined sugars are truly "empty calorie" foods, in that they essentially provide only calories, with no significant accompanying nutrition.

Whenever you begin to change a food from its natural state you start to sacrifice nutrients. Vitamins like A, C, and some members of the B-complex are partially destroyed by exposure to heat, light, and air, as are other substances like certain amino acids, the constituents of protein. Losses may be marginal as in freezing or juicing, or downright devastating as in deep frying, boiling, and high temperature baking or broiling, but by far the most drastic changes occur when entire parts of a food are removed as in the production of white flour, white rice, and refined sugars. What remains are vastly depleted foods that have lost much of their essential nutrition. Although a feeble attempt is often made to "enrich" white flour and rice by adding a few synthetic nutrients, they are still a long way from being natural foods by anyone's yardstick.

Vitamins and minerals are essential to life; this is an unavoidable fact of the universe. Just how much of each substance is needed for optimum health is a subject of heated debate among physicians, scientists, and self-styled nutritionists. Out of this confusion at least one thought impresses the common sense: since Nature has been in the business of recommending Minimum Daily Requirements for essential nutrients a lot longer than all of us, it seems reasonable to assume that a diet consisting of a variety of natural foods in amounts sufficient to maintain ideal body weight should contain sufficient vitamins, minerals, proteins, fats, carbohydrates, and any other mysterious elements we may as yet know nothing about. In other words, eat whole, natural, unprocessed food and you'll get all the nutrition you need.

Although it is definitely in a class by itself, alcohol has many of the same characteristics as refined sugar, and nutritionally it is similar to a refined carbohydrate, devoid of fiber and all other nutrients—a classic empty calorie food. Of course, alcohol does far more harm than any other refined carbohydrate, affecting principally the brain, heart, and liver in a most destructive fashion. Alcohol is the fourth leading public health problem in the United States, and anyone concerned with better health should sharply limit or eliminate its use.

Let's look at some simple figures. If Nature intends you to get 100 percent of your vitamins from 100 percent of your food, then getting say 20 percent of your daily calories from "empty" foods like sugar and alcohol means that you must get 100 percent of your vitamins from only 80 percent of your food. It's easy to see how as your consumption of refined foods increases, so does your vitamin deficit. Some people try to solve this problem with vitamin pills, but this is at best only a partial solution since vitamin supplements contain only the *known* nutrients. It is most likely that there are *unknown* nutrients in food which are life-supportive but which we have so far been unable to identify and synthesize.

The second, and possibly most important problem from a practical standpoint, is that refined carbohydrates are too quickly digested, making the experience of satiety too short-lived. For example, two people sit down to breakfast. One has a bowl of oatmeal with slices of fresh apple and a few raisins. The other has white bread toast with jam (primarily sugar) and coffee with sugar. Although the two may have taken in equal amounts of calories, our friend who ate the oatmeal will coast comfortably until lunchtime without hunger pangs, while the white bread guy will be looking for a snack in about two hours. The bottom line here should be obvious. The snack will add more calories, and if he snacks on refined food (which more than likely he will), this fellow will continue to need satisfaction on a more frequent basis than the person eating unrefined foods, especially unrefined carbohydrates. It's not hard to see that this style of eating will gradually lead to obesity. This is not the only cause of obesity, you should know. The more significant factor, "caloric density," will be discussed a bit later.

Salt

Salt has been justifiably indicted in at least one medical problem: hypertension, or high blood pressure. Salt attracts water and as the circulatory system retains water, the pressure on arteries increases. High blood pressure is a killer, no doubt about it, and everyone should take a close look at his salt intake.

The problem compound is sodium chloride, a combination of two essential nutrients, sodium and chlorine, and although both are needed by the healthy body, these needs are usually met by eating fruits and vegetables. Additional salt used in cooking or at the table should be strictly controlled. A healthy, natural food diet will provide about 0.5 gram (500 milligrams) of sodium per day, which is all you ever need regardless of your activities. You may safely take up to 3 to 5 grams (3000–5000 mg) but more is pressing your luck. If you eliminate your salt shaker and use a little salt in cooking only, you can stay within healthy bounds. The worst offenders are prepared and processed foods. Commercial catsup, mayonnaise, salad dressings, and other condiments are loaded with salt, and it is virtually impossible to maintain a safe balance of sodium using these foods regularly. Other foods high in sodium are meats, cheese, butter, margarine, eggs, and tuna fish. Three and a half ounces of bacon alone will put you over the 3 gram mark. If high blood pressure is a concern to you, you might invest in a cheap pocketbook salt guide to help you monitor your daily intake.

But what about sweating? If I'm out jogging in the blazing sun each day or working out at the gym, don't I have to replace all that lost salt? Actually, no. You really don't lose very much salt during sweating, and what little you lose is easily replaced by the natural sodium in fruits, vegetables, and grains. Even if you're running a marathon and sweating intensely for a prolonged period of time, the body implements its own natural survival controls and closes the gates at some point so that valuable minerals cannot pass out and you are ultimately sweating little more than pure water. Actually you wind up with a *higher* concentration of sodium in the body, since you lose more water than salt.[13] The danger inherent in marathon running is dehydration due to insufficient water intake during the run rather than the loss of electrolytes, the electrically charged mineral ions found in body tissues.

Fiber

An obvious component missing from white flour, white rice, and all refined sugars is what nutritionists call dietary fiber, and Grandma used to call "roughage." Fiber is a paradox. Although most is indigestible and non-nutritive, it is nevertheless essential. Fiber serves as a "buffer," regulating the rate of both digestion and assimilation. More critical, it stimulates the intestinal tract by producing larger bulkier stools which tend to move more efficiently through the system and are eliminated quickly and effortlessly. Anyone who has read the first six volumes of the *Encyclopedia Brittanica* while perched on the john knows the joys of a low fiber diet. Such a diet unfortunately produces more than mere inconvenience and discomfort. The low fiber regime has been indicted in a host of human maladies, including appendicitis, hemorrhoids, diverticulitis, gallstones, hiatus hernia, varicose veins, diabetes, elevated cholesterol and triglycerides, coronary artery disease, and, most significant, cancer of the colon, although all the evidence is not yet in on this. Good evidence shows that adequate fiber in the diet can lower serum cholesterol by 10 to 17 percent.

Since constipation seems to be at the root of all these problems, I feel it is essential that we understand this term. Many people consider themselves constipated only if they fail to have a bowel movement for two or more days, but consider themselves "regular" if they have a movement once a day. I believe this is incorrect. The healthy person on a healthy high fiber diet should probably have at least two major bowel movements a day. This is what we observe in wild animals as well as in groups of people living in "less civilized" areas of the world where traditional diets are still eaten. What is perhaps more important than the frequency of bowel movements is their character. A healthy stool should be large, soft, and well formed, in contrast to the hard little balls that usually emerge from those on a low fiber, high fat diet.[14]

Complex Carbohydrates

Carbohydrate is the perfect nutrient. The excess nitrogen in protein must be excreted, and so must the end products of fat utilization, but all carbohydrate is utilized. It is the food from which we derive our energy; it feeds our muscles and our brains. It is truly the basic fuel of the human body.

Sugars, even those found in fresh fruits, are *simple carbohydrates*. They are absorbed rather quickly, and although quite useful, do not have the sustaining power of the long-chain starches which we call *complex carbohydrates*. This is why a meal consisting only of fruit never seems to keep you satisfied very long. This is not to suggest that fruits are not desirable in the diet. They most certainly are, as they are excellent sources of readily assimilable vitamins and minerals; but although their carbohydrate content is valuable for short-term energy needs, a proper diet depends upon complex carbohydrates for continued energy production.

Refined carbohydrates behave more like simple carbohydrates in the digestive system. Their lack of fiber allows them to be broken down and assimilated too quickly, and sustained energy is not provided. The complex carbohydrate digests at a gradual pace, feeding glucose into the bloodstream at a steady rate, maintaining satiety for longer periods. The following is a list of typical complex carbohydrate foods, the type of food around which a healthy diet ought to center:

—all whole grains (brown rice, wheat, rye, millet, buckwheat, corn, barley, etc.)
—all whole beans
—all unrefined cereal products (oatmeal, cracked wheat, grits, flakes)
—breads made from whole grain flours (without added fat or oil)
—whole grain pasta

—potatoes and other root vegetables (carrots, turnips, sweet potatoes, etc.).

Add to these all fresh fruits and vegetables and a few nuts and seeds if you wish and you've got as close to an ideal diet as one can get in today's world. Such a diet would provide all the necessary nutrients in proper amounts, and allow your body to function at its optimum, affording it superior protection against most of the major degenerative diseases so prevalent in our society.

Chemicals

As one major chemical manufacturer has taught us at great expense, all life is derived from chemicals. This is wordsmanship, however; but lest I fall into their trap, let me say up front that when I use the word "chemical" I am specifically referring to those substances which are man-made, regardless of their "natural" derivation, and which find their way into our bodies through an increasing variety of channels. A pesticide, for example, like an organophosphate, which is derived from organic sources is not necessarily harmless to the human system, anymore than certain mushrooms which grow naturally from the Earth can be eaten freely and without fear of the consequences. For reasons I make no pretense of understanding, our Creator has made both harmful and beneficial plants available to us. It is up to us to use our intelligence to choose among them.

That potentially dangerous chemicals have infiltrated our environment is obvious to anyone who even occasionally picks up a newspaper. Those of us who take the time to read labels know that many processed foods contain artificial chemicals, some of which may have not been adequately tested. Of those tested, some have been preliminarily cleared for use (GRAS—Generally Regarded As Safe, the official government classification given to them), some will continue to be used while awaiting further testing, and a few have been linked to diseases. Nitrates are slowly being withdrawn from use in bacon, hot dogs, and lunch meats as a result of their apparent connection to stomach cancer. Polyvinylchloride shows strong links to cancer of the liver, and the list goes on. Some of these we can control and others we can't. Let us at least make an effort to eliminate the ones we can.

It is fair to say that there is as yet no overwhelming evidence that the chemicals being used in our foods as preservatives, colors, flavors, etc., are giving us cancer. It is also fair to say that there is no overwhelming evidence that they are not doing just that. What we have is more an information void than conflicting evidence. The discomforting truth is that most of our foods are laden with artificial substances about which we know virtually nothing—chemical time bombs implanted in our bodies which may explode into lethal growths twenty or twenty-five years later. Most cancer is not an inevitable fact of life. It is Nature's way of telling you you've broken the rules.

Why Eat Natural Foods?

Having read this far, you're probably getting the impression that in order to eat a healthy diet you're going to have to cut way back on or even eliminate many foods you have found pleasureable all your life. In addition, you'll have to learn to integrate new and possibly strange foods into your diet. This section will hopefully serve not only to summarize and expand upon the information preceding it, but also to offer you some strong incentive to give it a try.

As I see it, eating a natural food diet, foods considered natural according to our definition, will do the following for you: (1) reduce your chances of developing most of the major degenerative diseases which have become so common in our society; (2) help you to lose weight if you need to and greatly reduce the tendency toward becoming overweight, regardless of age; (3) increase your life expectancy, statistically speaking at least; and, (4) improve the quality of your daily life and extend a certain measure of youthful vigor into your later years. Let us consider each of these subjects individually.

Disease

Our natural food diet will be, by definition, considerably lower in fat than the typical Western diet. This will reduce your chances of developing fat-related diseases like atherosclerosis (hardening of the arteries), diabetes, heart disease, and possibly certain types of cancer.

The diet will also be high in fiber, and those diseases attributable to a deficiency of dietary fiber may therefore be viewed with far less concern. A natural high fiber diet may very well be your best defense against disease.

In fact, there is good reason to believe that a high fiber diet may even serve to protect us against environmental toxins coming into our bodies through drinking water or by way of the chemicals sprayed on fruits and vegetables. Laboratory animals given known poisons in certain dosages died when these poisons accompanied a low fiber diet, yet there was no effect on animals eating a high fiber diet.[15] Presumably the poisons were absorbed into the feces and eliminated before they had time to adversely affect tissues.

The optimal diet will consist of food of high nutritional value and all essential nutrients required from food will be plentiful. This will protect you from deficiency-related diseases and also eliminate the need for using costly vitamin and mineral supplements on a regular basis, although there may be periods of unusual stress or transient illness when use of these is indicated. Incidentally, if a little voice in the back of your brain keeps nagging you about something called vitamin B12, don't worry about it. It is discussed at length in Chapter 4.

Since processed and prepared foods will be eliminated or minimized, the diet will allow you to more carefully control your salt intake, thus lessening your chances of developing hypertension.

Finally, the diet will be as low as possible in the artificial chemicals so often found in processed foods, and although we can point to little hard evidence indicting these substances at this time, it is comforting to know you're on the safe side. Ten years from now when they say, "Oh, by the way, that stuff we've been putting in your salad dressing causes cancer. We're sorry, and we'll stop using it just as soon as our current supplies run out," you can breathe a little easier than others.

Obesity

All the statistics point to the same disturbing fact: far too many people in Western societies are overweight, often dangerously so, and as a society we are becoming more obese every year. Obviously our modern life-style, with its accompanying lack of physical work, is a great contributor, but many people who do hard physical labor or who exercise vigorously remain frustratingly overweight. Are we eating more? Perhaps, but the key seems to be not the amount of food taken in each day but the quality of that food.

We know that refined foods lack fiber and provide only brief satisfaction of hunger pangs, thus leading one to eat more often throughout the day—better known as snacking. This obviously leads to a greater total caloric intake and generously contributes to weight gain. Let me now acquaint you with a far more significant concept in the production of obesity—*caloric density*.

As the name implies, caloric density refers to the number of calories packed inside a given unit of food. Just as a cubic foot of cement will weigh more than a cubic foot of wood due to different specific gravities, so a cubic foot of cheese will have more calories than a cubic foot of lettuce. If we compare them by weight rather than volume we get the same effect. A pound of cheese will contain approximately 1700 calories, a pound of lettuce only 50. No doubt this difference is due partly to the amount of fiber and water in lettuce, and this is important; but it is due more to the fact that cheese contains a large amount of fat, and fat is itself a high density food.

You see, of the three major components of food—fat, protein, and carbohydrate—both protein and carbohydrate contain four calories per gram, while fat contains nine calories per gram, more than twice as much. So, the higher the percentage of fat in any given food, the more calories it will possess compared to the same amount of a food with less fat. Potatoes, which are largely carbohydrate, contain 279 calories per pound; while vegetable oil, which is 100 percent fat, has more than 4000 calories for the same amount.

Now, obviously these are extreme examples used to emphasize the point. I realize you are not apt to sit down to a big bowl of vegetable oil as you might potatoes, yet even the lesser differences which exist between routinely consumed foods in normal amounts, when totaled up at the end of the day, show that far more calories are taken in if the fat content of foods is not carefully monitored. Let's take a couple of examples.

A pound of mashed potatoes yields 340 calories (no butter, no milk), yet the same amount of french fries has 771 calories. You've essentially more than doubled your caloric intake with the same weight and much the same volume of food. Your stomach feels just as full, yet you've added an unnecessary 441 calories to your day's total. The difference is due to the vegetable oil or lard used to fry the potatoes. This is 100 percent fat, with little if any nutritional benefit.

Two cups of cooked brown rice, spiced up to taste and served with a salad will make a filling lunch. That pile of rice will provide about 350 calories. If you decided to eat cheese instead of rice along with your salad, you would only be allowed 3½ ounces of most types of cheese in order to equal the same number of calories obtained from the rice. How full are you going to feel after 3½ ounces of cheese? Not very, I would guess.

The examples could go on and on, but the point is clear. The more fat in your food, the greater the caloric density; the more calories absorbed, the more weight gain potential. The typical fast food lunch consisting of a cheeseburger, french fries, and a shake might net you 1500 calories or more, whereas an equally filling and far more beneficial lunch could be made up of whole grains and vegetables for less than 500 calories.

Weight control is like balancing your check book. To keep from getting overdrawn you must put in at least as much as you take out. To keep from losing weight you put in (eat) as many calories as you take out (burn up). Conversely, to keep from getting overweight you have to take out (burn up) as many calories as you put in (eat).

Now, an athlete training for the Olympics or planning to win the Boston Marathon can afford to take in 5000 or 6000 calories a day, so perhaps he need not worry about the food he eats, at least from the point of view of weight control. He should, incidentally, concern himself with what he eats, since exercise will do little to protect one from the ravages of a poor diet. But for the average person—the office worker and weekend jock—exercise usually equals greater hunger, and if that increased hunger is satisfied with the same high caloric density foods, the result will still be creeping obesity. The solution of course is to trim the fatty foods out of your diet, substituting unrefined complex carbohydrates wherever possible. This will enable the athletic and the sedentary alike to eat their fill and regulate their body weight more efficiently.

In case you haven't picked up on it by now, what I'm saying here is pure heresy and I would probably have been burned at the stake back in the days when the Atkins and Stillman diets ruled the empire. I'm saying that if you want to get thin and stay thin you should eat lots of carbohydrates—potatoes, brown rice, whole wheat bread, spaghetti—all those things you always thought were fattening. You don't believe me do you?

Carbohydrates have been the most maligned and misunderstood food in history,[16] and most of the confusion results from a failure to distinguish between simple and complex carbohydrates. When the good doctor told you to lay off the carbohydrates and lose a few pounds, he was thinking in terms of donuts, chocolate cake, and pancakes with maple syrup. These, if made with white flour, all contain simple carbohydrates, or at least behave the same way in the system. The actual carbohydrate contained in these foods is not by itself fattening; it's the fats that go along with it and the tendency of refined foods to digest too quickly and keep you hungry all day that cause weight gain.

If we switch to a diet centering around unrefined complex carbohydrates and are conscious of what we are adding to them, we are taking in comparatively few calories in each meal. This means potatoes without butter and sour cream, whole wheat bread made without oil and sweetener, brown rice without butter, whole grain pasta without cheese, and so forth; plus of course all the vegetables you can handle, and a reasonable amount of fruit.

An interesting experiment is worth mentioning here to drive home this point. Twenty-three young men were persuaded to eat two pounds of potatoes every day for three months. This equals about ten large potatoes, and as long as they consumed this quota each day they could eat anything else they wanted. By the end of the three months most of the men had actually lost weight.[17] Now, you need not go to such extremes, but the lesson should be apparent. The tendency of unrefined complex carbohydrates to fill up your stomach with relatively few calories makes them the ideal food for dieting and weight control. You still don't believe me do you?

Most people don't until they have tried it and seen for themselves, no matter how much sense the figures make to them. We have become so conditioned to believe that protein is good and carbohydrate is bad and that a high protein diet is the only sensible path to weight loss. In view of current knowledge we can see the shortcomings of these popular reducing diets. The high protein-low carbohydrate diet, with all its cottage cheese, hard-boiled eggs, and meat dishes increases the risks of developing all those conditions we now know to be associated with too much protein and fat. Besides all this, recent evidence has shown that high protein diets do not promote weight loss at all, and in fact encourage weight gain in the long run, probably by upsetting basal metabolism.[18]

A word of caution: I don't want to leave you with the impression that you cannot become overweight eating natural foods. What is "natural" may be subject to individual definition. Honey, for example, is not really an unrefined food. Although Man may not process it, the bees do. It is a concentrated, refined food and as such should be used sparingly. Caloric density is the most important concept, and it overrides the relative "naturalness" of any food at least with regard to weight control. Avocados, olives, nuts, seeds, peanut butter, dried fruits, and anything made with oil are all high calorie foods and must be moderated by those with a tendency toward weight gain.

Isn't It Expensive?

Second only to "the check is in the mail," the greatest lie of the 20th century may be that eating a natural food diet is too expensive. With most diets the amount of money you spend depends largely on the quality of food you buy. You may dine on filet mignon or chuck steak, lobster tails or codfish, and start a meal with caviar or Campbell's soup. With natural foods, however, a curious thing happens: the better your diet gets, the cheaper it is. If you simply want to continue the same basic diet you have but substitute a natural food counterpart for each processed and chemicalized product you buy, sure its going to be more expensive. Honey costs more than sugar, unrefined oils more than Mazola and granola more than Sugar Crunchies. And if you start snacking on nuts and dried fruit, you can bet they will cost more than Twinkies. But once your diet becomes "purer," focusing to a greater extent on fruits, vegetables, grains and beans, you'll find your weekly food bill dropping rapidly. A pound of brown rice will go a long way.

You'll eat less on a natural food diet too. Take a whole loaf of white bread and squish it together in your hands and you'll wind up with a lump of dough about the size of a baseball. It's not hard to see that you can easily eat half a loaf or more without feeling full. Try that with a good whole grain bread and you'll start to get the picture. Whole foods provide nutrition *and* bulk—bulk to give you the feeling of satiety before you overeat and bulk to keep your entire digestive and eliminitive system running efficiently.

Add to all of this, if you will, the savings a healthy person reaps in fewer trips to the doctor, less medicine from the drugstore, and fewer lost work days, and the financial effect becomes more evident.

Longevity and the Quality of Life

Will eating natural foods help you live longer? Research shows that Seventh-day Adventist men, who avoid tobacco and alcohol, and eat a natural vegetarian or low animal fat diet, in fact live longer by 6.2 years.[19] It would be unfair to attribute this increased longevity solely to the natural food diet, since non-smoking contributes at least half this effect. Nevertheless, the diet obviously is a significant contributor, and a sound diet generally leads to the adoption of other good health habits like non-smoking.

The important point is that a healthful diet and life-style provide a healthy active defense system, and the body can thus fend off environmental toxins and possibly even a small number of cancer cells better than a body fed a poor diet and engaged in a poor life-style.[20] Now, a gain of 6.2 years in a lifetime may not seem like all that great a reward for changing one's entire style of living. The real gain, however, is not so much longevity as in the quality of life during the later years. Another study showed that elderly people practicing good health habits exhibited vigor comparable to those thirty years their junior.[21] The point is simple: you can live to be seventy-five or eighty, crippled by osteoporosis, scarred by the surgeon's knife, drugged and senile, or you can live as *long or longer* but with the physical vigor and mental awareness of a person thirty years younger.

Q. *My husband and I could probably change to this type of diet without too much trouble, but our kids will fight us to the death. How can we win them over without a hunger strike?*

A. Subversion is the key. The logic of eating good food to help prevent coronary heart disease or diabetes does not appeal to the pre-adult mind. You have to get them to like the taste. The way to do this is to sneak it into their diet gradually so they don't know what's happening. As they become more accustomed to the taste and texture they will grow to like the diet. If you're used to serving white rice, mix in a small amount of brown rice. If you serve white pasta, throw in some whole wheat or spinach pasta with it. Make some homemade soups and put in beans, corn, and whole barley. Rather than go for a coarse, whole wheat bread right away, try a bread made with part whole wheat and part white or gluten flour. As they accept this, adjust the mix until the healthy food predominates.

Then there's always the "absent-minded shopper" technique. If you want to stop giving them the ritual ice cream after dinner, just "forget" to buy ice cream when it runs out. Offer them an alternative dessert. Don't worry, they won't pack their bags and leave home.

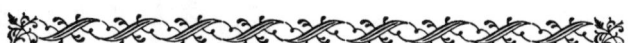

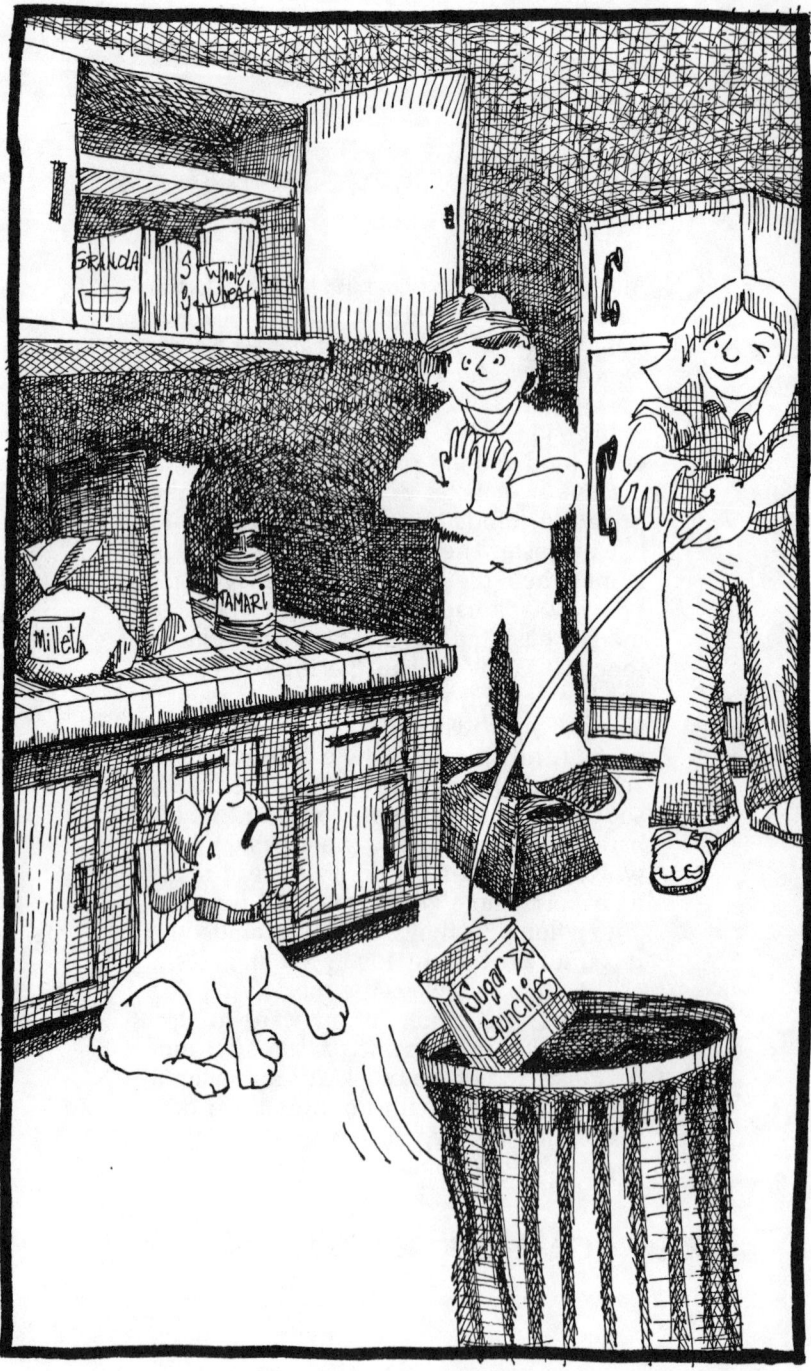

CHAPTER 2
Transition

If you've ever experienced a long airplane trip which put you through several time zones and perhaps a major climate change, you know its debilitating effects. You're tired, weak, constipated, and uptight, and it usually takes a day or two to adjust to the time change and even longer to the climate change. The fact is that organisms respond far more favorably to gradual than to abrupt changes. The human body is remarkably adaptable, but adaptation may have its side effects if it is required to take place too rapidly. This applies to diet as well, and if the change from a refined and processed food diet is to be successful it must be done gradually.

A number of factors suggest the desirability of a gradual transition. First, a person eating a refined food diet has a digestive system generally unaccustomed to bulk and fiber; his intestinal tract may be too narrow to handle it smoothly. People often experience severe cramping in this area because fiber is gas-forming and the colon needs to adjust to the expansion produced by this gas. The muscles which line the walls of your lower intestines may need some "breaking in." One does not run a marathon after spending a month in bed.

Second, there is the cleansing process to deal with. The human body likes to clean itself out when it has been polluted with foreign substances. As soon as you start eating wholesome food exclusively, your body will begin to aid Nature to purge it of toxic residues, since it is no longer overloaded with them. If the change to pure food is gradual, so will be the cleansing, and you will experience only the benefits not the process, of this house-cleaning. If you try to leap too quickly into a pure diet, however, you may endure some unpleasant side effects: weakness, headaches, strong body odor, skin blemishes—all possible indications of internal reconstruction taking place, perhaps a bit too quickly.

Last, the taste buds may need a little time to readjust. If you're accustomed to heavily salted, sugared, greasy foods, your taste receptors may be so overstimulated that pure, natural food will taste bland and boring. This may discourage you and induce you to give up on the whole project—"I'd rather take my chances with cancer and heart disease than live my life eating boring food." Sound familiar? I remember when I first gave up using salt. Everything tasted like newspaper for two weeks. Then for the first time in my life I began tasting vegetables. A salad became a bowl of different tastes rather than an indistinct mound I managed to eat only after it had been drenched with a half bottle of some salty, sugary dressing.

I know thousands of people who have made the transition to real food, and without exception they now thoroughly enjoy their diet in every way. I don't want you to give up, which is why I cannot overemphasize the importance of a gradual change.

The entire transition may take anywhere from six months to a year depending on just how bad your diet is now and how far you want to go toward an optimal diet. Although each individual must tailor this transition to his own physical and psychological needs, the following may serve at least as an educational guide.

Step 1: Read the labels on all the prepared products you are using at home. Eliminate or substitute natural foods for all those containing additives like chemical preservatives, emulsifiers, stabilizers, artificial colors and flavors. If you can't pronounce it, don't eat it.

Step 2: Reduce red meat consumption to three times a week. Eat more fish and poultry. Take the skin off poultry and throw it out. Try an occasional vegetarian meal.

Step 3: Toss out your salt shaker and begin to use less salt in cooking. Watch out for prepared products containing salt.

Step 4: Eliminate white flour and cut back on sugar. Use only whole grain breads and products made from whole grains. Choose products made with sweeteners in the natural state, e.g., fruits and fruit juices.

Step 5: Choose lightly steamed fresh vegetables over boiled, and eat more raw green salads.

Step 6: Reduce meat consumption further. Try to base your meals on white fish and vegetarian foods. Be careful not to go overboard on dairy products and eggs during this period.

Step 7: Eliminate refined sugar totally, and begin to cut the consumption of all "sugars," including honey. Satisfy your sweet tooth with dried fruit.

Step 8: Eliminate meat for all but special occasions or entirely. Use white fish and skinned poultry sparingly. Keep eggs, cheese, milk and milk products to a minimum. Have more vegetarian meals centering around whole grains, beans, potatoes, and vegetables.

Step 9: Eliminate all sugars. Choose fresh fruit over dried fruit for sweets.* Reduce direct use of salt in cooking and seasoning to a minimum. Eliminate all prepared products, "natural" or otherwise, which are high in salt, sugars, or fats.

Step 10: At this point your diet should consist of fresh raw fruits, fresh raw or lightly steamed vegetables, whole grains, beans (if you like them), small amounts of milk (preferably nonfat) and cheese (preferably nonfat), eggs occasionally, only if you must, some fish (not shellfish) and skinned poultry, and only small amounts of meat, if desired.

If you make it to Step 10, you're fairly close to an ideal diet. Some may want to go a bit farther and eliminate all flesh foods, eggs, and dairy products. This is quite safe and in fact desirable from all current indications in the medical literature. A diet consisting solely of fresh fruits and vegetables, along with whole grains, will satisfy every nutritional requirement for a healthy human being.

As we shall see, some people go even farther toward "purity" by eating only raw foods or only fruit, but such extremism is not recommended.

---

*Diabetics or hypoglycemics may have to limit even fresh fruits.

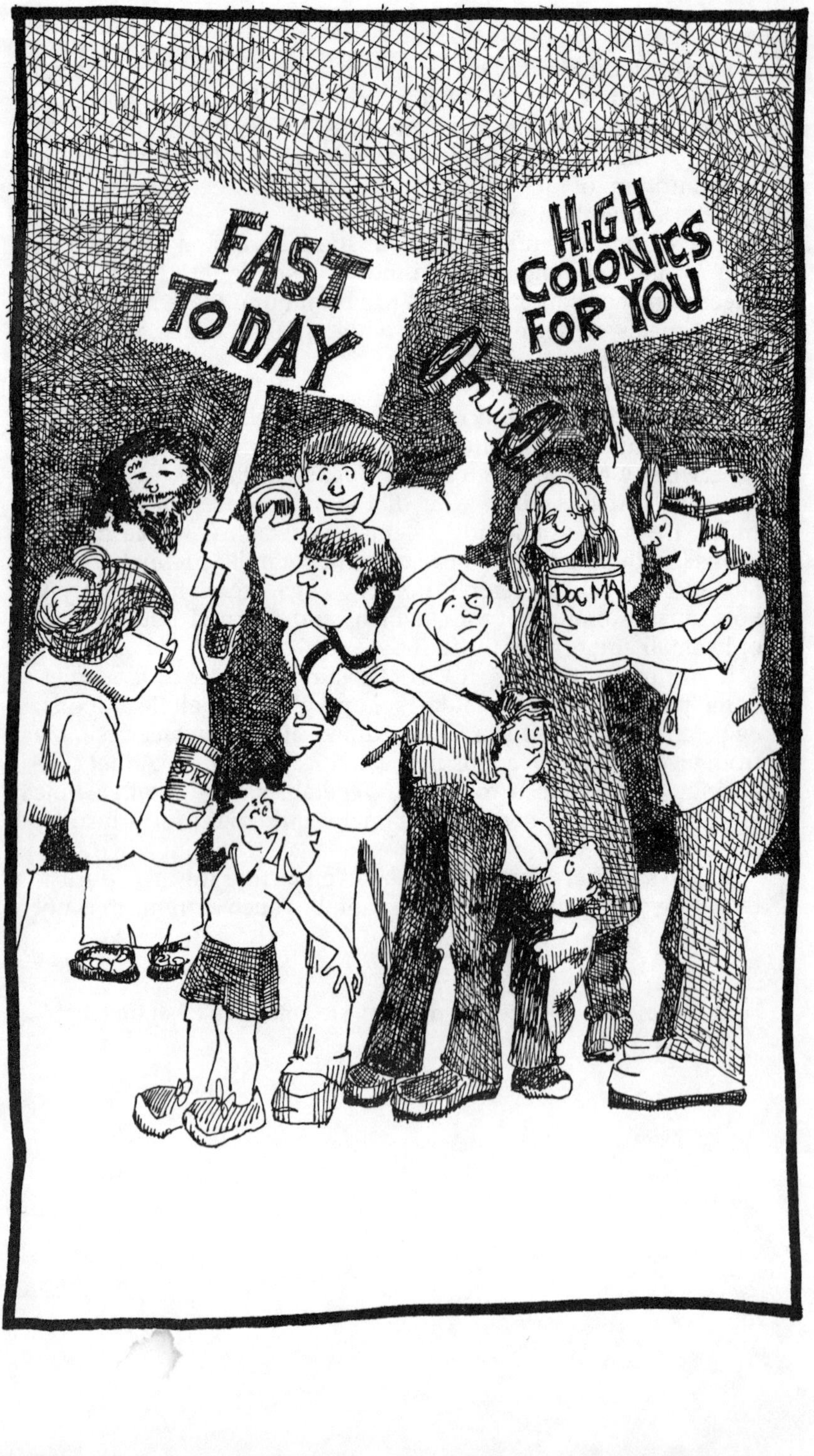
FAST TODAY
HIGH COLONICS FOR YOU
DOG MA

CHAPTER 3
On the Fringe

If you're going to start hanging around natural food stores, reading the books, and talking to the people who work and shop there, you're going to hear a lot of strange talk about radical diets, fasting, cleansing, food combining, and so forth. So that you may understand the jargon being thrown around, I have included this little crash course in the fringe elements of nutrition. Some of these disciplines embrace basically sound ideas which have positive applications for many people, perhaps yourself, while others are forms of extremism which, although they may someday prove to be valid, are as yet unacceptable to the mainstream public and possibly dangerous to followers.

It is wise to be wary of the proselytizer. He wants to draw you into his personal philosophy of diet more often for his benefit than for yours. His strange and radical ideas may seem romantic and attractive but could be physically destructive. He may not practice what he preaches but use others as unknowning guinea pigs. In some instances his faddism or fanaticism may be a result of serious psychological disturbance.

It is best to look for a certain natural logic in choosing a dietary path. Who am I and how do I fit into the general scheme of Nature? What are the foods available to me and what is known about them? What are the pressures, physical, social, and pychological, that I must deal with in deciding a direction? A diet consisting entirely of fruits and nuts may be fine for someone living in a tropical jungle, free of the stresses of urban life, but how do I relate to this?

Lacto-ovo-vegetarian—eats eggs, milk and milk products, and all plant foods, but does not eat flesh foods, i.e., meat, fish, or poultry. This is the most common form of vegetarianism and that practiced by major religious groups like Seventh-day Adventists.

Lacto-vegetarian—eats milk products and plant foods but excludes eggs and flesh. This diet, like the lacto-ovo-vegetarian regime, may be chosen for health or moral reasons, the individual feeling that the slaughter of animals is wrong. The lacto-vegetarian may consider an egg a potential life and therefore as sacred as the living animal. This is common among the religions and philosophies transplanted from India.

Strict or total vegetarian—eats no animal products whatsoever, i.e., no milk, eggs, or flesh. Strict vegetarians are often cautious about "hidden" animal products such as gelatin capsules (made from animal connective tissues) or vitamins containing fish liver oil.

Macrobiotics—a diet based upon that eaten by a group of Japanese monks renowned for their superior health. The macrobiotic diet centers around cooked grains (mostly brown rice), cooked vegetables, and miso soup, with only a small amount of raw salad and fruit, and little if any meat. There are various stages in macrobiotics, each one progressing to a more grain-centered diet. The ultimate and most infamous of these is Macrobiotic Diet #10, which is only brown rice. That's it folks, brown rice—breakfast, lunch, and dinner. Great for people who hate to make decisions. The #10 diet is usually misunderstood, and often the entire doctrine of macrobiotics is maligned on the basis of this one relatively unimportant aspect. The total brown rice diet was developed not as something to live by but rather as a short-term diet for purposes of body cleansing and meditation. It is apparently easier to meditate when you have nothing to look forward to but another bowl of brown rice.

On the whole, a sensible macrobiotic diet can be fairly well balanced, although on the surface it does seem to be low in certain nutrients, particularly vitamins A and C. The high sodium content of miso should be another concern.

Vegan—strict vegetarian with strong philosophical convictions that prohibit using any animal products in his life-style, even if not connected with diet. Some vegans, for example, will not own or use any products made of leather, fur, or animal parts of any kind. This is a very difficult credo to live by, since animal by-products are used so extensively in industry. The rubber that goes into automobile tires and tennis shoes, for example, contains animal fat products. In general, the vegan philosophy overrules nutritional common sense. Many vegans subsist on tea and white biscuits and thus are rather unhealthy.

Fruitarian—believes that only fruit is proper food for Man. Some have the philosophy that vegetables have life just like animals, and it is as morally wrong to take the life of a carrot as to take the life of a cow. Fruits fall freely from the tree when ripened and eating the fruit has no effect on the life of the tree. Philosophical beliefs aside, the all fruit diet can be healthy providing a wide variety of fruits are eaten. Fruits contain all the required vitamins, minerals, fats, carbohydrates, and proteins in sufficient amounts so long as enough calories can be obtained. Herein lies the difficulty for most people. It is extremely hard to acquire enough calories on a fruitarian diet to maintain a healthy body weight. A rapid and significant weight loss usually occurs within the first month of the diet, and although the loss is small and gradual during subsequent months, it nevertheless continues until the person is genuinely endangered by caloric malnutrition, or more properly under-nutrition.

Getting enough calories is not impossible, just difficult. One must be prepared to eat tremendous amounts of fruit or lots of high calorie fruits like olives and avocados, and generally limit physical activities considerably so as not to demand more calories. Often fruitarians include nuts in their definition of fruit, and this appears to be a far more sensible regime.

Sproutarian—subsists exclusively on sprouted grains, sprouted beans, and sprouted vegetable seeds. Good luck.

Breatharian—more a theoretical and philosophical ideal than a practical reality. The belief is that a person can attain such a high state of purity and spiritual development that he can subsist totally on air and sunshine. Very economical.

Raw foodist—never cooks food because he believes that cooking destroys critical enzymes present only in the raw state. Raw foodists are usually strict vegetarians living on raw fruits, vegetables, sprouted grains and beans, nuts, and seeds. Some, however, use raw milk, raw eggs, even raw meats, especially organ meats. Brain salad anyone?

There is no evidence that plant enzymes serve any useful

purpose in the human system, but, regardless, the notion that raw food is superior to cooked is, for the most part, nutritionally sound. However, I would avoid raw eggs (see Chapter 14), and would be very careful with raw meat as it is infamous for harboring parasites and various other dangerous organisms. Also, foods like grains, beans, and potatoes, which contain complex starch chains, are relatively undigestible in the raw state. This, in my opinion, represents a serious flaw in the raw food philosophy.

Cooking destroys nutrients, no doubt about that, and raw foods will always contain more vitamins, minerals, and proteins. On the other hand, cooking also makes some nutrients more *available* to the body. Carrots, for example, are loaded with vitamin A (in the form of carotene), but it is locked up in little cellulose packets which our digestive system is unable to break down, so as much as 50 percent of this vitamin load may pass through the body unabsorbed. Light cooking breaks down the cellulose, making the vitamins accessible for absorption. Of course, overcooking will not only break down the cellulose but also destroy much of the vitamin, so a certain amount of discretion is called for. The raw foodist can overcome this problem either by chewing his food unmercifully in order to mechanically break down the cellulose or by pureeing carrots and other tough vegetables like coarse leafy greens in a blender or juicer.

Mucousless diet—avoidance of so-called mucous-forming foods, which include just about everything except raw fruits and vegetables. This is primarily used as a "healing" diet when sickness is present or great deterioration of the body is suspected due to poor diet. The mucousless diet usually involves fasting and colon cleansing as well.

Protein complementing—based on the fallacy that vegetable proteins are incomplete and must be mixed together in proper combinations and proportions in order to yield total proteins which the body can use. Rice, for example, was considered to be an incomplete and inferior protein until mixed with beans, which "filled in" the weak spots in the protein and made it useful. Modern research has shown that a complete protein at each meal is not necessary and that today's vegetarian in the United States need not concern himself with complementing proteins (see Chapter 4).

Food combining—a system developed by the American National Hygiene Society's leader, Herbert Shelton. Although somewhat complicated, the general idea is that different classes of foods interfere with each other's complete digestion, since each requires special digestive processes. One should not, for example, mix fruits and vegetables at the same meal, or proteins and starch, or even sweet fruit and acid fruit. The results of poor food combinations are said to be faulty digestion, poor absorption of nutrients, putrefaction in the stomach and intestines, foul smelling stools, and flatulence. That's enough to get you voted out of your neighborhood fast.

Of those who have endured the discipline of "proper food combining," some swear by its positive results while others report it to be intolerably boring. It is fair to say that medical evidence in support of the theory is not overwhelming, and it is conceivable that many of the experienced results are psychosomatic. There is growing feeling, however, among those who study nutrition and digestion seriously that we should all work toward eating less complicated meals. Variety is important in the *overall* dietary picture, but simplicity should be a goal within each meal. Those who suffer from indigestion and flatulence would do well to try to avoid too many different foods at one meal.

Fasting—technically, fasting is the abstinence from all food for a period of time. Nutrition writers use the term differently, however, and speak of *juice fasts*, where only fruit and/or vegetable juice is taken, *fruit fasts*, where only fruit is eaten, or *water fasts*, where water is the sole "food."

The goal of fasting is usually a combination of purification and weight loss. The principle is that once the body stops receiving food or certain foods it will begin to cleanse itself by breaking down stored fats and thus releasing various toxins which have been hiding in these fats. The toxins are released into the bloodstream along with other products of fat breakdown and hopefully shuffled out of the body fast enough to prevent them from doing any harm.

You may hear about persons accomplishing remarkable physical feats while fasting. This is almost always in reference to juice fasting, which provides a good level of carbohydrates for energy production. Since fruit and vegetable juices contain all the necessary nutritional elements except dietary fiber, this is not as surprising as it first seems.

If the idea of an occasional fast appeals to you, you should know that of the three types, only the fruit fast may be recommended without sincere criticism. Although juice fasting is common, there may be a danger involved. It has been shown that sugar considerably decreases the ability of the white blood cells to engulf germs. This happens even with orange juice due to its high natural sugar content, and the effect lasts up to 5½ hours.[1] Eating whole fruit, with its fiber intact, decreases the rapidity with which the sugar is absorbed and eliminates or at least minimizes this effect.

Extended water fasts can be more troublesome. Often, many stored toxins are thrown into the system, resulting in an undesirable imbalance in the body. Also, there is a saturated fat problem. When you are digesting yourself, which is precisely what you are doing after about three days on a water fast, you are digesting *animal fat*. After all, you *are* an animal and your stored fat *is* animal fat even though you may have eaten vegetables to get it. So, suddenly you have a bloodstream full of saturated fat, which will cause your oxygen uptake to decrease dramatically and possibly lay down permanent fats in your arteries.

A simple fruit fast, eating as much fruit as you desire for one or more days, will accomplish the basic goals of fasting: (1) the rate at which fruit is digested and eliminated will give your system a sort of "cleansing"; (2) the lack of fats, concentrated proteins, and complex carbohydrates will give the system a "rest"; (3) you'll probably lose some weight; and (4) the discipline will be good for you.

My feeling, however, is that if you want to "clean yourself out," you should do it the same way you "dirtied yourself up," that is, slowly and gradually. Just get on a pure natural food diet and let your body take care of the cleansing process slowly and painlessly. It may take a few years but this is the safest way. If quick weight loss is your prime objective, fasting is typically only a temporary solution. Most people overindulge themselves after a fast and rapidly gain back their weight.

Colonics (colonic irrigation)—this is the cleansing craze taken to its logical extreme. Operated largely by chiropractors and naturopathic doctors, colonic centers are cropping up all over the place. These centers offer a program designed to "rebuild" the colon through fasting, the ingestion of some type of intestinal cleanser (usually herbs and certain seeds like psyllium and flax), and regularly scheduled colonic irrigations, whereby a long tube is inserted into the rectum, winding its merry way into the colon, and releasing water and/or oxygen, thus forcing out the fecal matter. The process is based upon the premise that a poor diet will distort the colon and cause all sorts of nasty things to get caught up inside it. Once this ancient fecal matter is released and washed out by irrigation, the person is rejuvenated and ready to begin a pure diet designed to prevent this from happening again.

Although I don't doubt that colonic irrigation is a useful technique under certain unique circumstances, like a totally blocked colon, its current widespread use among basically healthy people for the purpose of cleansing themselves has no sound medical basis. First, the premise upon which colonics have become popular—that pockets are formed in the colon where fecal matter is trapped and remains due to a faulty diet—is not supported by those who have examined large numbers of colons. Except in the cases of bedridden persons who are unable to change their body positions often and a few others, bowel physiologists who have inspected literally thousands of human colons simply do not report this fabled condition.

At the very least, colonics are a waste of money for most people. If constipation is your problem, the switch to a grain-centered diet will take care of you quickly. If it's cleansing you want, the natural food diet is the only sensible answer.

Are colonics harmful? Well, they will of course wash out electrolytes and certain colonic bacteria responsible for producing important body nutrients, and if done too often you could produce weakening of the intestinal muscles and even, in extreme cases, dependency upon the technique. As I see it, however, the real danger in colonics is the growing tendency for people to consider them as panaceas. There is no substitute for a proper diet—not vitamin pills, not fasting, and certainly not colonics. You don't binge on donuts, pizza, and ice cream and then simply drop into your neighborhood colonic irrigation center and have your sins washed away, and expect to remain healthy for life. The human body was not designed to operate that way, and all you're doing is buying time.

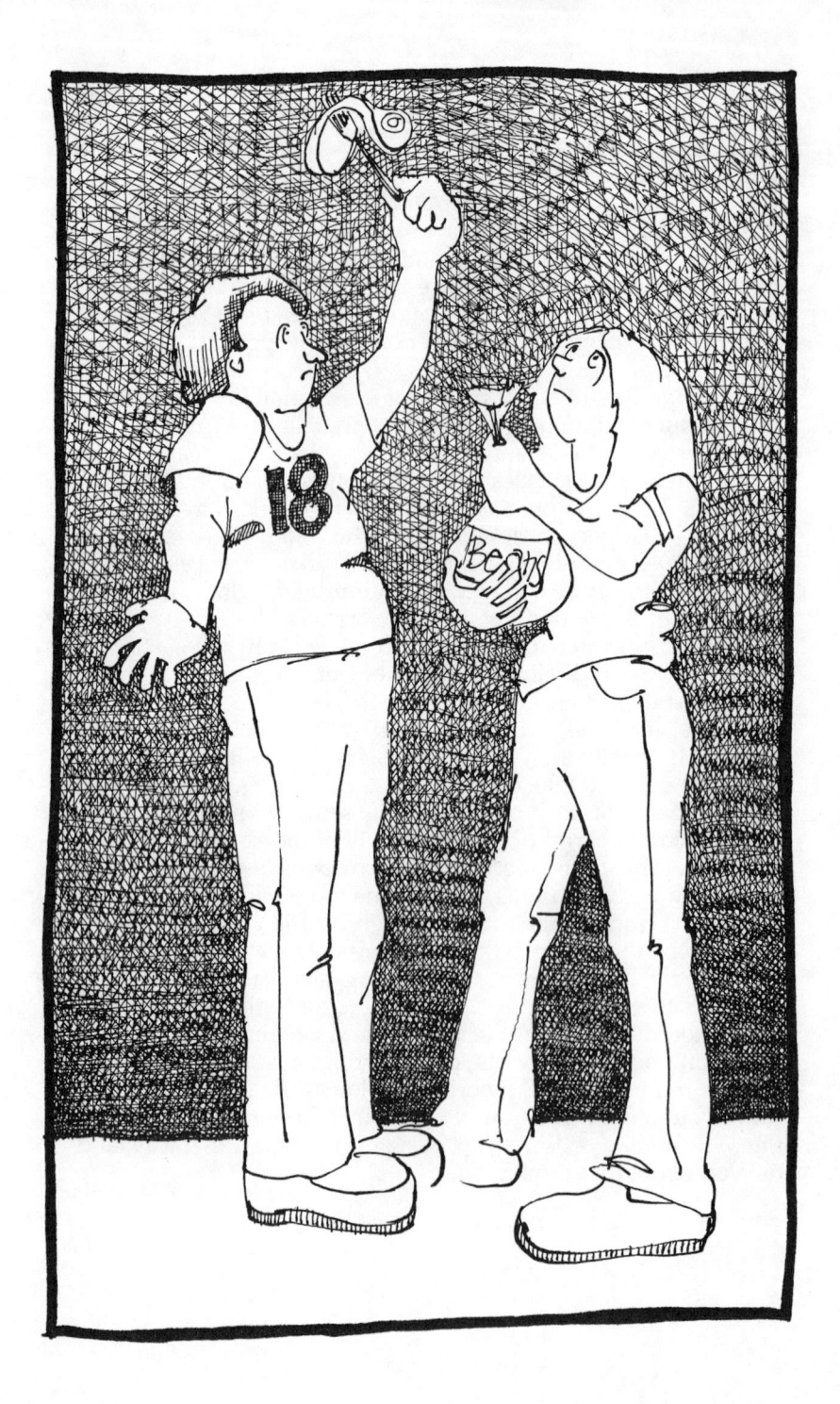

CHAPTER 4
The Protein Problem

Whether the idea of eventually becoming a vegetarian is attractive or absurd to you, the fact is that the change from unhealthy to healthy foods is almost always accompanied by a shift away from a meat-centered diet. This lessening importance of meat in your life comes about for two reasons: one, because you will learn more and more about the unhealthy aspects of meat consumption, and two, because as your body becomes "cleaner" from eating better foods, your desire for meat will decrease significantly. You will become more sensitive to your body, which intrinsically knows what's good for you.

One of the challenges you must be prepared to face as you begin to move toward a more plant-centered diet is that inevitable question: "But where will you get your protein?" This question will come from your friends, your relatives, and often from those you assume to be experts on matters of diet and health. If your own family doctor is typical, he will be thoroughly uneducated in nutrition, and will not have kept up with the medical literature pertinent to that field. Thus, he may express sincere and well-intentioned concern over your deviation from the dietary norm. If he is really uninformed, he may suggest that giving up meat is dangerous. If he is slightly enlightened he may tell you that you can survive without meat only if you eat plenty of milk, cheese, and eggs for protein. He'd be a real flaming liberal if he explained that it is even possible to derive adequate protein from plant sources providing your meals are carefully designed to insure that all the essential amino acids (constituents of protein) are present simultaneously. This would necessitate considerable study and planning on your part, he might add, and probably wouldn't be worth it.

If the above three bits of advice were posed in the form of a multiple choice question, the answer would be: (D) none of the above. All currently accepted research and expert opinion agree: the protein problem is not really a problem at all, except perhaps for the meat, dairy, and egg industries, for which it is a profit problem.

What is protein?

Let's take a close look at this protein business and see just what we know about it today. First, we should understand exactly what protein is. There is a group of biochemicals, essential to life, known as *amino acids*. These are relatively simple organic compounds with funny names like lysine, methionine, tryptophan, and phenylalanine. Depending on who is doing the counting, we need about twenty-two of these amino acids to stay alive and well. All but nine are produced quite naturally and routinely in the human body. The nine (ten in the case of children) must be obtained from the environment in the form of ingested food. These are known collectively as the Essential Amino Acids (EAA's), and any food containing all nine EAA's in proper proportions is called a *complete protein*. You may also hear some talk about *inferior* and *superior proteins*. The egg, for example, is reputed to be a superior protein, since the EAA's are in exceptionally good balance. Many vegetable proteins are deemed inferior because one or two EAA's are low in proportion to the others. As we shall see, this distinction is arbitrary and meaningless from a practical point of view.

Once nutritionists progressed beyond the type of thinking that led us to believe we would die without eating meat, or at least using milk and eggs in abundance, they began talking about something called *protein complementing* or amino acid balancing. The idea was that two so-called inferior proteins, like corn and beans, each high in certain amino acids but low in others, could be mixed together to produce a superior protein, since each would complement the other's weaknesses. In this way, plant foods could produce protein comparable to that in meat, and the vegetarian need not lie awake at night in dread of developing a protein deficiency. A paperback entitled *Diet for a Small Planet*, by Frances Moore Lappé (Ballantine, 1971) emerged from this great discovery, and taught millions how to correctly mix their brown rice and soybeans.

The concern over proper protein complementing was based on the assumption that for a protein to be well utilized by the body, all the component amino acids had to be present in the same meal. In other words, you had to eat the corn and beans together, not at separate meals, or it just wouldn't work. We now know that none of this is true. Research has shown that the body indeed has lots of amino acids available at all times, and foods low in certain of these are readily complemented from stored supplies, presumably in the form of cells sloughing off the lining of the stomach and being metabolized into their useable components, and from various digestive juices.[1] In other words, the amino acids from all of your foods—from carrots, bananas, rice, bread, broccoli, and oatmeal—are absorbed into your body and combined whenever necessary with other amino acids taken in at different times (amino acids now in the form of digestive juices, stomach cells, etc.) producing a complete protein.

How much protein do we need?

Having established that protein is reasonably simple to obtain, the next logical question concerns the quantities needed on a daily basis. The Recommended Daily Allowance for protein is about 10 percent of your calories, but this has been purposely overestimated and most experts agree that 5 percent is adequate. This means that a person eating 2000 calories per day needs only 100 of those calories from protein. Since there are 4 calories to each gram of protein, about 25 grams per day is fine. Now, armed with these vital figures, you could of course spend hours pouring over all those exciting food composition charts to determine if your protein needs are being met. Forget it. The simple truth is that as long as you eat whole, unrefined foods, you'll get enough protein providing you get enough calories. In fact, it is quite impossible to design a diet consisting of whole unprocessed fruits, vegetables, and grains that is protein deficient as long as it meets your calorie needs. In other words, if you're getting enough calories to maintain your body weight, and those calories are coming from whole foods in a reasonable variety, you're getting enough protein.[2]

This relationship between calories and protein remains valid regardless of your level of physical activity. Protein has nothing to do with energy or stamina. Whether you are a marathon runner, a power weight lifter, or a monk, your protein needs remain at 5 to 10 percent of your calories. Naturally the person who exercises vigorously will require more calories in his diet, and hence will get more protein if the percentage is maintained, but protein above this level is unnecessary and unhealthy. Body builders are often obsessed with the misconception that they need huge amounts of protein to build muscle bulk, which is "torn down" during workouts. This is a fallacy. The amount of muscle building that can take place in a 24-hour period is minute, and a normal protein intake will easily provide all the raw materials necessary. Body builders who take in excess amounts of protein are risking kidney failure and softening of the bones in later life.

What is wrong with eating meat anyway?

Despite the fact that Man has obviously consumed meat during certain eras, there are many who feel this was merely a temporary adaptation necessary for the survival of the species under exceptional environmental pressures. The evolutionist believes that when the lush forests which were the natural habitat of Vegetarian Man began to disappear with the dawning of the Ice Age, we were forced into a hostile environment where there was little left to eat other than animals, and perhaps even each other. For this and other reasons, there is considerable question about whether meat is a natural food for Man, or for that matter even a beneficial food. The creationist, of course, accepts the simple biblical account that man in his original state was a vegetarian.

A look at the biological structure of Man and a typical meat-eating animal strongly suggests that we have no business eating meat. The run-of-the-mill carnivore, like a cat or dog, has a digestive system roughly three times the length of its body. This allows ingested flesh to enter the system, have its nutrients absorbed, and be pushed out quickly, before the by-products of its deterioration within the body begin to cause trouble. Man, on the other hand, has a digestive system more like *twelve* times the length of his body, and a lower fiber food like meat spends entirely too long winding its way through the labyrinth, putrifying along the way, and creating nasty compounds like neutral sterols and other substances which have been strongly linked with cancer of the bowel.[3]

Nutritionally, meat stacks up very poorly. It is far too high in saturated fat and totally devoid of fiber and carbohydrate, two major dietary components, and there are simply not enough vitamins and minerals in meat to override its nutritional drawbacks.

Another danger of meat is what Man has added to it. Literally hundreds of chemical compounds may find their way into your steak dinner: hormones, antibiotics, preservatives, and artificial colorings and flavorings, many of which, like nitrates and growth hormones, have been in the Top Ten of the Cancer Hit Parade for years.

Even economically, meat is a losing proposition. It is second only to sugar and sweets as the poorest buy nutritionally. There is nothing in meat you cannot get from other foods, far more cheaply and safely.

OK, I'm convinced, but what about milk and eggs?

Cow's milk is a perfect food—for calves. Goat's milk is great for little goats and human milk is great for little humans. All natural mammals are raised on their own mother's milk until a given age, after which they take no more milk for the rest of their lives. Humans should be no exception to this rule of Nature. Cow's milk is totally different from human milk: it differs in the quality and quantity of protein and fat; it differs in carbohydrate and vitamin and mineral content. And these differences are not so small and insignificant. The total nutritional picture of cow's milk is as different from that of human milk as a cow is different from you, which makes rather good sense when you think about it.

One of the most obvious and striking differences shown in the table on the next page is in the percentages of protein. Human milk contains a mere 6 percent protein, and this is the sole source of protein for the developing infant in its most intense and demanding growth period. Never again will the human body increase its weight so rapidly and require so much protein, yet a food with only 6 percent does the job perfectly. So why, after our child has done so beautifully on a 6 percent protein food, do we insist he drink each day a quart of cow's milk, containing 3½ times the amount of protein?

With regard to fat, note that although human milk is higher in fat, less than half is saturated, while almost two-thirds of cow's

Nutrient Values for Cow's and Human Milk

	100g. Cow's Milk	100g. Human Milk
Calories	61	70
Percent of calories as protein	21.6	5.9
Percent of calories as fat	49.3	56.3
Percent of fat that is saturated	62.3	45.9
Percent of fat that is unsaturated	32.3	49.3
Percent carbohydrate	30.6	39.4
Sodium	49mg	17mg
Calcium	119mg	32mg
Phosphorus	93mg	14mg
Vitamin C	0.94mg	5mg
Vitamin A	126 I.U.	241 I.U.*

*International units.
Source: U.S. Dept. of Agriculture Handbook no. 8-1.

milk is saturated fat. It is known that polyunsaturates are particularly important for developing infants, since linoleic acid (found in polyunsaturates) is essential for proper formation of the nervous system.

It is also curious that the calcium level of human milk is roughly one-fourth that of cow's milk. This points out the absurdity of the drink-your-milk-for-strong-bones syndrome. How do all these breast fed babies manage to develop normal bones and teeth with such paltry amounts of calcium? Obviously, our obsession with calcium needs reexamining.

Finally, take a look at the low sodium level in human milk, and the high amounts of vitamin A and especially vitamin C. This is Nature's natural food for humans during their most important stage of growth, and observing its composition should give a clearer insight into Nature's idea of nutritional needs.

If we use human milk as a reference and assume that adults require sodium, for example, on an equal weight basis with infants, we can see that 5 grams of salt per day should fill adult needs. This could mean having no salt shaker on the table, using no highly salted foods, such as potato chips, and using little meat, but using a little salt for cooking.

Although there are a number of nutritional and digestibility problems with milk and milk products, the main one is too much fat. Expressed as percentage of calories made up by fat, milk is 49 percent, cottage cheese is 41 percent, and cheddar cheese is a whopping 76 percent fat. The developing infant needs lots of fat for its emerging nervous system, but once this process is complete, fat requirements are considerably lower, and excess fat becomes problematic.

More important than the absolute amount of fat in the diet is the quality of that fat. A diet high in fats of any kind, saturated or unsaturated, is unwise, yet it is the saturated variety that appears to do the most damage. The typical Western diet, consisting of 40 percent fat, mostly saturated, has been indicted in a number of killing diseases, including breast cancer, colon cancer, and atherosclerosis.[4] In the last, fats and cholesterol are gradually laid down in the linings of the arteries like rust inside a pipe. As it builds up over the years the blood vessels become more and more constricted until finally one closes completely, blocking blood flow to a vital organ like the heart or brain, and it's all over, baby.

The intake of more than small amounts of milk, milk products, and eggs (with 72 percent of their calories as fat), and meat of course, puts the individual at great risk of developing closure of the arteries, regardless of age. Autopsies on many young soldiers killed in Korea showed severe narrowing of the major blood vessels in American men with an average age of only twenty-two, while a similar examination of young Japanese soldiers showed no such atherosclerotic formations.[5] And a large number of epidemiological studies have shown that in countries where the use of milk, eggs, and meat is low, so is the occurrence of heart disease, cancer, and many other fat-related maladies.[6] Wherever the Western-style high-fat diet is introduced to other peoples, so are these diseases.

What about fish?

Fish has a couple of redeeming features, but many of the same problems as meat, milk, and eggs. Choosing carefully among the many types of fish available and restricting your consumption to once or twice a week will minimize some of these, however. Let us consider some of the pros and cons of fish.

PRO: The saturated fat content is not high.
CON: Cholesterol levels are equal to beef and lamb in most scaly fish, and exceptionally high in shellfish.
CON: Fish are high in long-chain polyunsaturated fatty acids (see Chapter 5), with many double bonds which tend to

oxidize more rapidly, forming peroxides, which some scientists look upon as carcinogenic.

CON: Fish are quite high in protein and present the same problems as other high protein foods (excessive demands on the kidneys, increased urinary excretion of calcium drawn from the bones, uric acid production). However, if fish are eaten only occasionally, this should be less important in the total picture.

CON: Fish are deficient in dietary fiber. The problems associated with low fiber foods can be avoided by eating fish in small amounts along with other high fiber foods (as the Japanese do).

PRO: Fish are not usually treated with chemicals like growth hormones or nitrates as meat often is.

CON: However, they may absorb toxins from polluted waters and for this reason should be selected with care. Those from lakes, rivers, and streams defiled by the waste products of industry and society should be avoided, as should scavenger fish (like shellfish), which feed on garbage near ocean shores.

Another type of fish you should consider avoiding are the large ocean going species like tuna, shark, and swordfish. They accumulate large amounts of toxins and heavy metals in their fatty tissues because they are at the end of long "food chains," which means that they have eaten smaller fish which in turn have eaten even smaller fish and so on down the line. In each case the larger predator inherits all the toxins of its prey. This may put you in mind of the "mercury scare" of some years ago. Press coverage fell quickly and the public seemed to just forget about it, but the mercury didn't go away. It continues to be stored in the fatty tissues of fish and in your tissues when you eat them.

CON: Fish develop cancer, and that cancer may be passed on. One percent of fish in Canadian waters and four percent in the Fox River basin (awash with chemical wastes from Chicago) have tumors, and it has been shown that cancer can be transmitted from one animal to another, even in a different species, by eating the flesh of the diseased animal.[7]

All things considered, fish does not stack up as the most desirable food for Man. Since, like all animal foods, it has no special, hard-to-get nutritional benefits, it seems sensible to eat it only in small quantities as a taste treat, and even then to select it carefully. The small, white-fleshed ocean varieties, preferably those which feed in seaweed beds and not on garbage—snapper, sea bass, sole, cod, butterfish, and others—seem to be the safest bet.

If I don't eat any of these foods, won't I develop a B12 deficiency?

Historically, it was believed that B12, a compound essential for blood formation and growth, was exclusively an animal product, and anyone daring to eliminate flesh, milk, and eggs from his diet would eventually develop *nutritional macrocytic anemia*, the result of vitamin B12 deficiency.

As more and more people turned to total vegetarianism as a means of achieving superior health, it was assumed that a veritable epidemic of B12 deficiencies would emerge. It didn't. Except for a few cases, persons forgoing animal products plodded happily along without ever developing B12 related anemias.[8] Why?

First, vitamin B12 requirements are extremely low. Whereas almost all other recommended nutrient allowances are measured in *milligrams* (thousandths of a gram), B12 is measured in *micrograms* (millionths of a gram), so miniscule are the needs.

Second, the body has so large and efficient a storage capacity for B12 that if you had no dietary source whatsoever, your supply would last five to seven years.

Third, a few non-animal foods contain B12 in abundance. Although they are not yet what you might consider common table foods, they are nevertheless available to those who feel they want insurance. *Tempeh* and *miso* are among them, and these are discussed later.

Last, all of the above is probably irrelevant since it has been long suspected, and recently demonstrated, that B12 is produced and absorbed quite naturally in the healthy human digestive system by normally occurring bacteria.[9] I suspect that the multitude of bacteria in the mouth cavity are also producing B12 all day long and it is routinely being swallowed and assimilated.

So the spectre of nutritional macrocytic anemia is, for most of us, of historical interest only. The person committed to avoiding all foods of animal origin need not concern himself with taking B12 supplements, unless he is among those rare individuals whose systems fail to produce and absorb this vitamin.

Toward an Ideal Diet

As our knowledge of human nutrition broadens, we begin to see a clearer picture of what may be the ideal diet for Modern Man. All indications are that animal foods, be they flesh, milk, or eggs, are not well suited as food for humans. They appear to be too high in fat, too high in protein, lacking in carbohydrate and fiber, and generally polluted with toxic and potentially carcinogenic chemicals, either by design or circumstance. There also seems to be nothing special about animal foods from a nutritional standpoint. They possess no known nutrients that we cannot obtain easily from plants, more safely and more economically. Experimental studies fail to demonstrate any advantage to eating animal foods, in fact quite the contrary. Vegetarians have lower blood pressure, less obesity, less risk of heart disease and cancer, and great vigor and longevity. They exhibit greater stamina when compared to meat eaters in endurance contests, and there is hardly an athletic pursuit on this planet that does not have outstanding participants who are vegetarians, including weight lifting. Add to this, if you will, the fact that the largest and strongest animals on Earth are, and always have been vegetarians (elephants, horses, etc).

We have previously discussed the problems inherent in simple sugars, white flour, white rice, alcohol, and all other refined and highly processed foods. "Empty calorie" foods have no place in the ideal diet. Carbohydrates must be of the complex "as grown" variety, untampered with by Man and his technology.

The evidence is also gathering against high fat diets regardless of the type of fat consumed. Saturated fat is, of course, still the major villain, but unsaturated fats appear to have safety limits as well. Neophyte vegetarians all too often consume huge amounts of nuts, seeds, and peanut butter, partly out of naive concern over getting adequate protein and partly to satisfy their "fat tooth," so to speak.

The ideal diet then is low in *all* fats (saturated fats in particular), low in protein, and high in natural carbohydrate; it is plant-centered rather than animal-centered. Concentrated simple sugars, such as those found in honey, molasses, and dried fruits, are restricted.

Nathan Pritikin, director of the Longevity Center, recommends the 10–10–80 diet, which translates to 10 percent fat (mostly unsaturated), 10 percent protein, and 80 percent natural carbohydrates. Others feel that more linoleic acid is needed in the diet than can be obtained from a 10 percent fat regime, and suggest a 20–10–70 diet—20 percent fat (largely from polyunsaturated oils), 10 percent protein, and 70 percent carbohydrates.

The exact figures may not be all that critical, but they are indeed a far cry from the average American diet consisting of 45 percent carbohydrate (mostly refined and severely deficient in fiber, vitamins, and minerals), 15 percent protein, and 40 percent fat, and highly saturated.

So, what's left to eat. The ideal diet would consist exclusively of fruits, vegetables, whole grains, and products made from whole grains. Beans may be used if you like them, but they are not essential.

Now, before you throw this book away in disgust, it is fair to say that the ideal diet, like all ideals, is meant to be *approached* rather than attained. It is not an all-or-nothing proposition. You do not necessarily have to completely give up meat, cheese, fish, poultry, eggs, nuts, seeds, honey, and so forth. What you can do is strive to get as close as possible to the ideal within the bounds of your own personal, social, and psychological needs. Each individual must seek his own *balance*. If giving up all animal foods makes it impossible for you to carry on your business lunches without disapproval from your peers, then don't give them up—but, make up for it at home with lots of whole, high fiber foods. On the other hand, you might find that ordering a vegetarian lunch makes for interesting conversation, and you may just end up saving your boss or client from a heart attack. And if a cocktail with your friends is an important part of your social life, denying yourself this small pleasure may be more harmful psychologically than the drink is physically. In other words, the first principle of nutrition education is: it's not what's on the table but what's on the chair that counts. When your mind and attitude see the light, then make the dietary changes.

Enough philosophy. If you have read this far and are still interested, read on—the balance of this book contains the practical information you will need to design and maintain any level of healthful diet you choose.

Scores of excellent natural food cookbooks are available, and I have no desire to compete with them. However, a few recipes are included at the end of each chapter, mainly so that you can put the practical information into perspective by seeing how it fits into a real meal. Also, a small amount of nutritional data are included so you can compare the values of various foods. You need *not* labor over these charts and tables to tally up your daily quota of this vitamin or that mineral. Just eat and be merry— Nature will do the rest.

Q. *How about pregnant women—don't they require extra protein?*

A. Pregnant women need more calories; and if they eat a whole, natural food diet, more calories will automatically equal more protein. All you're doing is eating extra food for the developing fetus. That extra food should be no different in quality and variety than your normal diet.

Think of it like building a house. If you decide to build a five-room house, you will need a certain amount of lumber, nails, glass, paint, etc. If you later want to add a sixth room, you'll need just 20 percent more of the same materials, not different materials. Growing a child inside you is like adding another room onto your body. Just give it the same food you feed yourself and it will grow just fine.

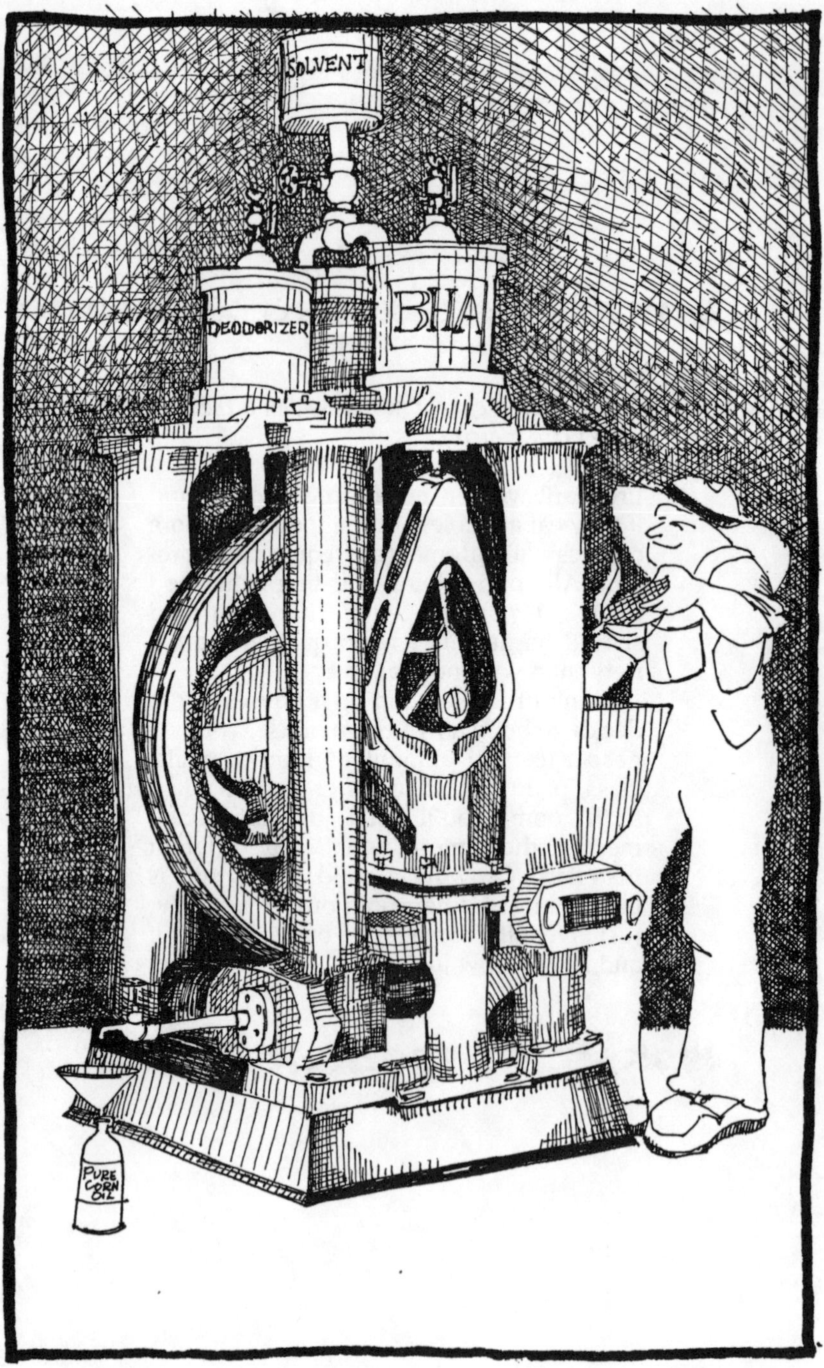
SOLVENT
DEODORIZER
BHA
PURE CORN OIL

CHAPTER 5
Oils

What Is Fat?

When we talk about fat in foods we are essentially talking about a substance composed of a number of *fatty acids:* stearic acid, oleic acid, palmitic acid, linoleic acid, linolenic acid, and so forth. Each fat is made up of some proportion of fatty acids, and the relative amounts of each type of fatty acid determine the character of that fat. Pork fat is lower in palmitic and stearic and higher in oleic and linoleic acids than beef fat, for example. The word "fat," as it is used throughout this book, refers simply to any substance composed of fatty acids connected to a glycerol, whether of animal or vegetable origin. Oil, whether it comes from a soybean, an olive, an almond, or a sunflower seed, is made up of molecules consisting of three fatty acids connected to a glycerol, and is therefore a fat.

Saturated and Unsaturated Fats

Broadly speaking, edible fats may be divided into two classes: saturated and unsaturated. In order to understand just what this means, let me introduce you to just a tiny bit—I promise you no more—of biochemistry.

The following is the molecular structure of linoleic acid, a fatty acid your body needs to maintain good health.

$$H-\underset{\underset{H}{|}}{\overset{\overset{H}{|}}{C}}-\underset{\underset{H}{|}}{\overset{\overset{H}{|}}{C}}-\underset{\underset{H}{|}}{\overset{\overset{H}{|}}{C}}-\underset{\underset{H}{|}}{\overset{\overset{H}{|}}{C}}-\underset{}{\overset{\overset{H}{|}}{C}}=\underset{}{\overset{\overset{H}{|}}{C}}-\underset{\underset{H}{|}}{\overset{\overset{H}{|}}{C}}-\underset{}{\overset{\overset{H}{|}}{C}}=\underset{}{\overset{\overset{H}{|}}{C}}-\underset{\underset{H}{|}}{\overset{\overset{H}{|}}{C}}-\underset{\underset{H}{|}}{\overset{\overset{H}{|}}{C}}-\underset{\underset{H}{|}}{\overset{\overset{H}{|}}{C}}-\underset{\underset{H}{|}}{\overset{\overset{H}{|}}{C}}-\underset{\underset{H}{|}}{\overset{\overset{H}{|}}{C}}-\underset{\underset{H}{|}}{\overset{\overset{H}{|}}{C}}-\underset{OH}{\overset{}{C}}=O$$

Each carbon (C) atom is capable of forming a maximum of four *bonds* with other atoms, each line (−) in the diagram representing one of these bonds. Note that in some cases the carbon atom has bonded with hydrogen (H) atoms on three sides and with the next carbon atom in the chain. But at some points, where you see two lines (=), the carbon has failed to unite with a hydrogen and instead formed a *double bond* with its neighbor. Lacking a hydrogen at each available location is a state called *unsaturation*. Linoleic acid then is an *unsaturated fatty acid*, and since these double bonds appear more than once, it can be further defined as a *polyunsaturated fatty acid*. If only one double bond were present, as in oleic acid, it would be known as a *monounsaturated fatty acid*.

The next diagram shows the structure of stearic acid.

$$H-\underset{\underset{H}{|}}{\overset{\overset{H}{|}}{C}}-\underset{\underset{H}{|}}{\overset{\overset{H}{|}}{C}}-\underset{\underset{H}{|}}{\overset{\overset{H}{|}}{C}}-\underset{\underset{H}{|}}{\overset{\overset{H}{|}}{C}}-\underset{\underset{H}{|}}{\overset{\overset{H}{|}}{C}}-\underset{\underset{H}{|}}{\overset{\overset{H}{|}}{C}}-\underset{\underset{H}{|}}{\overset{\overset{H}{|}}{C}}-\underset{\underset{H}{|}}{\overset{\overset{H}{|}}{C}}-\underset{\underset{H}{|}}{\overset{\overset{H}{|}}{C}}-\underset{\underset{H}{|}}{\overset{\overset{H}{|}}{C}}-\underset{\underset{H}{|}}{\overset{\overset{H}{|}}{C}}-\underset{\underset{H}{|}}{\overset{\overset{H}{|}}{C}}-\underset{\underset{H}{|}}{\overset{\overset{H}{|}}{C}}-\underset{\underset{H}{|}}{\overset{\overset{H}{|}}{C}}-\underset{\underset{H}{|}}{\overset{\overset{H}{|}}{C}}-\underset{\underset{H}{|}}{\overset{\overset{H}{|}}{C}}-\underset{OH}{C}{=}O$$

In this case all bonding locations on each carbon atom are filled. The chain is considered saturated and this is a *saturated fatty acid*.

Now, all foods which contain fat contain both saturated and unsaturated fatty acids, but in varying proportions. Milk fat, for example, is quite high in saturated but low in unsaturated fat. Safflower oil is low in saturated and high in unsaturated fat. In general, animal foods are higher in saturated fat, and vegetable foods are higher in unsaturated fats, although this is not without exception. Coconut is extremely high in saturated fat, the highest in fact, but most fish are quite low in saturated fat and high in polyunsaturates.

Saturated fat is usually solid at room temperature—hard white fat that causes cholesterol to accumulate inside your circulatory system and eventually closes off arteries entirely. Although the mechanism by which this sequence of events occurs is yet unclear, studies of populations continue to confirm that people who have diets high in saturated fat (i.e., lots of fatty meats, eggs, and full fat dairy products) have significantly higher risk of heart disease and a number of other degenerative diseases. For this reason, it has been suggested by both independent nutritionists and government committees that we all seek to limit our intake of saturated fat.

Unsaturated fat, be it monounsaturated (like olive oil) or polyunsaturated (like corn oil), is liquid fat. There is no evidence that unsaturated fat causes cholesterol to accumulate in the arteries as does saturated fat, yet oils have their own complications and should be used sparingly. These are discussed more fully at the end of this chapter.

Hydrogenation

So what about Crisco and Spry? They say vegetable oil on the can yet they are solid white stuff. Are they just hard oils? In a sense the answer is "yes," they are hard oils, but what has happened here is that an unsaturated oil or fat has been transformed into a saturated fat by a process known as *hydrogenation*.

Remember our little single and double bonds between carbons in the diagrams of fatty acids? Well if you take a polyunsaturated oil and bubble hydrogen through it under pressure and in the presence of a metal like nickel, which acts as a catalyst (stimulates reaction), the double bonds are broken and hydrogen atoms are then bonded to all the available locations on each carbon. The previously unsaturated fat is now a saturated fat, and is referred to as a *hydrogenated fat* or *hydrogenated oil*. There is no reason to believe that some of these hydrogenated fats will behave any differently than ordinary saturated fats in your bloodstream. In other words, eating a food containing hydrogenated fat will have many of the same negative effects as eating a food naturally high in saturated fat. This is important to keep in mind when you read labels if your goal is to limit saturated fat.[1]

In actuality, oils are not *fully* hydrogenated, since that would result in fat too hard to use conveniently. In order to produce a stable fat which is still soft enough to work with, oils are only *partially hydrogenated*. The percentage of saturated fat is quite high though, so don't be mislead into thinking that a product listing "partially hydrogenated palm oil," is somehow not all that bad. If that phrase rings a bell, you've probably been reading a few labels lately. Many products, including some sold in health and natural food stores, contain "partially hydrogenated palm or soy oil," or "one or more of the following partially hydrogenated oils: cottonseed, palm, soy." Hydrogenated oils are easier to work with particularly in baked goods and candy manufacturing, and they sustain less spoilage than liquid oils.

All this translates into lower operating costs and higher profits, so the choice of hydrogenated oil is tempting to a producer.

The Manufacture of Oils

The labels found on bottles of oil often include terms that may be confusing to the consumer—words like "cold pressed," "mechanically pressed," "unrefined," and "unbleached." To understand these terms and their significance to health, we need to know a little about how oils are manufactured.

First the seeds, nuts, or beans that are the source of the oil are cleaned and hulled mechanically. Next, one of two processes takes place. In one, the cleaned source product is steamed (up to 250° F for cottonseed, and as low as 110° F for safflower) and then pressed in a high pressure *expeller*, which will heat it up to between 140° and 160° F, pressing out the oil by "squeezing" mechanically. At this point the oil may be simply filtered to remove large particles and bottled. This *unrefined mechanically pressed* or *expeller pressed* oil is the most desirable in terms of nutrient content, although it will retain a distinct taste and odor which may not appeal to those who are accustomed to bland deodorized oils.

In the alternative process, the cleaned seeds are rolled into flakes and treated with a solvent like hexane which acts to extract the oil chemically. Hexane is a petroleum derivative, and residue from it may remain in the oil. Following extraction, the oil will be distilled to evaporate excess water, and if it is bottled at this stage it will be considered "unrefined," but not "pressed." If it is to become a refined oil, it will pass through a number of steps involving degumming, treatment with alkali, bleaching, and deodorizing, which almost totally destroys all nutrients and produces a tasteless, odorless oil so familiar to those who purchase the commercial supermarket brands. Preservatives like BHA, BHT, or polysorbate 80 may also be added at this point.

Label Reading: 101

Oils sold in natural food stores often carry impressive looking labels that use all sorts of pure-sounding descriptive terms. Let's look at some of these and see what they actually mean, if anything.

Cold Pressed

The original cold pressed oil was produced by an old fashioned screwdown press. This process did not produce heat sufficient to destroy the nutrients, and the result was as pure a product as could be obtained. Cold pressing left a great deal of oil in the source residue, however, making it economically unappealing to large manufacturers. To resolve this problem, high pressure expellers were designed to more efficiently remove the oil from its source. These machines, however, generate a good deal of heat, enough to raise the oil temperature to 150° F or more. Clearly, this is not a "cold pressed" oil. *Whole Foods* magazine, which has become a highly respected watchdog of the natural foods industry, did extensive research and interviewing on the subject of cold pressed oils and concluded, by implication at least, that the term is patently false and misleading and should be dropped from labels if we are to fairly represent our products. There is no such thing as a cold pressed oil on the market. Companies that recognize and respect this fact are now changing their labels to read "mechanically pressed," "expeller pressed," or simply "pressed." All of these terms clearly distinguish these oils from those extracted by chemical solvents.

Unrefined

As shown before, unrefined or "crude" oil is bottled immediately after extraction and filtering, and does not proceed through the refining, bleaching, and deodorizing stages. The advantages of unrefined oils are the retention of important nutrients like vitamins A, E, and K, and the absence of residues from chemical solvents or additives. Unrefined oils have definite and varied tastes and odors which they impart to whatever food they are used in. Safflower oil is quite mild and soybean or peanut rather strong. These are not bad tastes, mind you, just distinctive.

In addition, unrefined oils smoke more readily when cooked, tend to solidify when refrigerated, and are inclined to get rancid faster than refined oils, particularly those with preservatives. But if you like the taste and learn to store them properly, they are by far the better buy due to their nutrient content and purity.

All oils sold in health and natural food stores are not necessarily unrefined. Hain, for example, is one major company bottling both refined and unrefined oils. As a rule, light-colored, clear oil without sediment is refined. Companies like Arrowhead Mills, Erewhon, and Westbrae offer unrefined oils of excellent quality. These oils are darker, with a thick murky sediment on the bottom that should be shaken into the oil before using.

Unbleached

Commercial oils are run through clay or charcoal to remove pigment. This involves temperatures up to 250°F, and any oil billing itself as unbleached will not have been subjected to this process or its associated heat.

No Cholesterol

Cholesterol is exclusively an animal product, and therefore all vegetable oils are cholesterol-free. Don't be mislead into thinking that only oils labeled "no cholesterol" are free of it. This information is included on a label only to inform those looking to avoid cholesterol in their diets, and as an advertising ploy.

Rancidity

A major problem with oils and foods containing oils is that they tend to go rancid. Technically, rancidity is called *oxidation*, and it is the result of oxygen molecules from the air combining with unsaturated fatty acids. The more unsatured the oil, the more readily it will oxidize to become rancid. Unfortunately, rancidity may mean a lot more than just stale-tasting food. There is growing opinion that rancid oils in food may be a prime cause of stomach cancer. For this reason, I strongly recommend that you take special care in storing your oils. Oil should never be left out, even unopened, for any length of time, but should be refrigerated. Some, like soy, peanut, and olive, may solidify under refrigeration but this is harmless. Oil that is left exposed and used over and over for deep frying, as in fast food outlets, is highly suspect, and any person on the road to better health should avoid such places.

Rancidity may occur even in an unopened bottle, especially if the oil was exposed to the air for some time before bottling. At least one company, *Arrowhead Mills*, is now doing something called *nitrogen flushing* to their bottled oils. This involves forcing nitrogen into the bottle after the oil is in and before it is capped. Nitrogen, a harmless component of the air we breathe, displaces the oxygen, forcing it out, and therefore leaving nothing to induce rancidity.

If you suspect an oil is rancid, the test is a definite "stale" smell and a burning sensation in the back of the throat a few moments after swallowing even a small amount.

Types of Oil

Practically every edible nut and seed contains a significant amount of oil, and depending on cost and availability, each may or may not be used for producing oils on a large scale. In addition, at least two grains, corn and wheat, and two legumes (soybeans and peanuts) are used for oils. Let's look first at the common oils used in cooking and in salad dressing, and then at some "exotic" oils, which although sometimes used as food, are more often in cosmetics.

Corn Oil

Most of the popular refined oils you buy in supermarkets are made from corn, it being relatively cheap to manufacture and high in polyunsaturates. Unrefined corn oil has a deep amber color and a distinct odor and taste. Corn oil is high in vitamin E, which protects against rancidity, and it is therefore considered a reasonably stable oil.

Soy Oil (Soya Oil, Soybean Oil)

Here is another good polyunsaturated oil, commonly used in baked goods, but almost always after being refined, since the unrefined oil has a strong taste that will dominate any food you put it in. Soy oil is light brown, with lots of gooey sediment. It is the most widely used oil in the U.S., and in fact accounts for two-thirds of all the oil used here.

Safflower Oil

Derived from the seed of a plant grown in California and Arizona, safflower oil is the darling of the natural foods industry. The polyunsaturate craze of cholesterol-conscious America has made safflower oil, the oil highest in those precious substances, a hero. This very quality, however, also makes safflower oil especially prone to rancidity, and it should be carefully protected. It is not advisable to use it for high temperature cooking, as deep frying, since the rate of oxidation is much increased. One would expect it to contain more vitamin E than corn oil since it is so high in polyunsaturates, but it does not.

Sesame Oil

This is the oriental favorite for stir-fry or wok-style cooking. Only a small amount is used, just enough to coat each chunk of food and seal in the nutrients. It is also an excellent salad oil, but like safflower, not recommended at high temperatures.

Sunflower Oil

Something of a newcomer on the scene, sunflower oil is gaining popularity, particularly on the commercial market. Second only to safflower oil in its degree of unsaturation, it also has a fairly light taste and odor, and so lends itself well to salad dressings. But it too is not recommended at high temperatures.

Peanut Oil

Like soybean oil, unrefined peanut oil has a taste you won't forget—all through your meal. It is generally used for cooking, especially in Indonesian dishes.

Olive Oil

Here is the crème de la crème of salad and cooking oils, and the price reflects it. Olive oil is not especially high in polyunsaturates, being right in the middle, and for that reason many consider it a "safe" oil. Safe in the sense that it is low enough in polyunsaturates to be stable in the presence of oxygen and not high enough in saturated fat to be considered a health problem if used in moderate amounts. It is made up primarily of the monounsaturated fatty acid, oleic acid, which tends neither to raise nor lower blood cholesterol levels. In Crete, where the people use as much fat as we do, they have only one-tenth as many heart attacks. This is probably because 80 percent of their fat is from olive oil.[2] Most people, however, prefer olive oil for one reason only, the taste, and it definitely is in a class by itself. Olive oil makes everything taste Mediterranean, and for most of us that's a pretty nice taste.

Olive oil is pressed from the fruit, the pit, or both. If pressed exclusively from the fruit, it is called *virgin olive oil*, and the best olive oil is labeled "100% virgin unrefined."

Palm Kernel Oil

You most likely won't find this in a bottle on anyone's shelf, but chances are you've eaten plenty of it in your lifetime. It is an oil very commonly used in candies, cakes, cookies, and confections of all kinds. Its high degree of saturation (85 percent) makes for a texture which lends itself well for use in coatings on candies, etc. Palm oil contains 39 percent palmitic acid, the most palmitic acid of any food, and this is the common fatty acid that tends to raise blood cholesterol.

Coconut Oil

The extreme of saturated oils (91 percent), with very few polyunsaturates (2.5 percent), coconut oil is also used extensively in confections and in cosmetics as well. Some cultures use it freely as a frying oil, but it is not recommended as an edible due to its highly saturated nature. Studies even show that oils used in moisturizing creams and suntan lotions may be absorbed and digested through the skin.[3]

Cottonseed Oil

Another of those "mystery" oils used in manufactured baked goods and confections, it is often labeled simply "vegetable oil." Since it comes from the seed of a plant which is ordinarily sprayed heavily for boll weevils, I am inclined to view it suspiciously. Also, at 25 percent saturated fat and 22 percent palmitic acid, it is unsuitable for those striving to avoid heart attacks.

Blended Oils

A few companies market products which consist of a blend of oils, usually soy, safflower, peanut, and something exotic like walnut oil or a small amount of olive oil for taste. These are pretty much to be considered gimmicks, and have no special nutritional advantage.

Exotic Oils

Some manufacturers bottle low popularity oils like pumpkin seed, apricot kernel, avocado, walnut, flaxseed, and rapeseed. These are sometimes used in salads (walnut) or in cooking (apricot), but more often applied topically to the skin in the belief that they have some rejuvenating effect on those tissues. "Natural" beauty books abound with cosmetic concoctions using unusual oils guaranteed to bring youthful elegance to that aging face in the mirror.

Wheat Germ Oil

I've left wheat germ oil for last since it is a special case. Wheat germ oil is not used functionally, that is to say, not in cooking or in salads, but is prized as a supplement, due to its relatively high vitamin E content. Whether or not vitamin E is of any great value to the human system is a subject of great debate, but since it is found in small amounts in many natural foods, nature probably put it there for a reason. In the center of the wheat berry is the germ, which consists largely of this valued oil. The oil is extracted, either by expeller pressing techniques or by chemical solvents, and bottled for sale, at around $7 a pint. Users of wheat germ oil take it straight from the bottle or mix it in drinks or with their regular salad oil. Personally, I'd rather eat the wheat and get my vitamin E as Nature offers it.

Some people give wheat germ oil to their dogs or horses to improve the appearance of their coats. However, if an animal's coat is lackluster, it is most likely due to a deficiency of linoleic acid, and this could be improved with any oil and a lot less expensively than with wheat germ oil.

Selection and Storage

Again, oils should be refrigerated after they've been opened and exposed to the air. Before that, you take your chances. When you buy an oil, subject it to the smell and taste test. If you are certain it's rancid, take it back, or throw it out if you're the kind of person who doesn't like taking things back, but by all means, don't use it. Before you jump to conclusions about rancidity, however, bear in mind that unrefined oils smell quite different from Wesson or Mazola, and if that's what you're used to, you might easily mistake the strong odor of an unrefined oil for rancidity. Also, do your store a favor—don't open up the oil on the shelf and sniff it. If you put it back after opening it, it will surely spoil. The best test is taste; that burning sensation in the back of the throat is a dead giveaway. Personally, I would be inclined to favor the nitrogen packed oils, since they give you a little edge on oxygen infiltration.

Occasionally, you will find stores selling oils in bulk, from big 55-gallon drums, the oil being dispensed through some sort of spigot system like those used to dispense soft drinks. There are only two ways oils can be kept fresh under these circumstances: the barrels of oil must be kept under refrigeration and only the dispensers left out in the store; or the entire system must be flushed with nitrogen and all the oxygen therefore displaced. With only nitrogen in the system, refrigeration is unnecessary. If your store sells bulk oils, ask them about their system. I'd be inclined to pass if neither refrigeration nor nitrogen flushing was being used.

On Oil in the Diet

Recent studies suggest that not only should we all take a critical look at the amount of saturated fat in our diet, but also at the *total* amount of fat, saturated or unsaturated. Although certain oils known to be high in polyunsaturates appear to have some therapeutic value in lowering blood cholesterol levels, there are still many drawbacks to the use of oil in general. Let us consider what we know at this point.
  1. Large amounts of certain oils, corn oil, for example, tend to cause gallstones,[4] but large amounts of olive oil, with its high percentage of monounsaturates (oleic acid), does not have this effect.
  2. Some laboratory studies on animals have shown that a diet high in polyunsaturates produces more cancer.[5] Whether it is the oil per se or some change that takes place in the oil is not yet clear. We know that oil oxidizes rather easily to form substances known as *peroxides*, and some scientists believe these to be carcinogens.

3. Even though unrefined oils may contain a few nutrients, they are still for the most part empty calorie foods, and for this reason should certainly be limited in one's diet.

Rather than look at a lot of scientific research and horror stories, let's instead ask one simple question: "Is oil a natural food?" By our definition, even the purest, most unrefined oil would not qualify, since nutritionally oil bears little resemblance to its source food. Soybeans, for example, are a wealth of vitamins, minerals, protein, carbohydrates, fat, and fiber. Yet soybean oil is just fat, 100 percent fat, retaining only small amounts of the fat soluble vitamins like A, E, and K.

If we were to obtain our oil only in the context of whole, natural foods, how much would nature allot us? The latest available figures (1980) show that the average American consumes almost 21.4 pounds of salad and cooking oil per year.[6] Try to imagine how much unprocessed food we would have to eat in order to obtain this much oil. To see how absurd this is, let's take the example of corn and corn oil. The average person might put two tablespoons of corn oil on a salad. This will amount to 252 calories and 28 grams of fat. In order to get that same amount of oil by eating fresh corn, you would have to eat twenty-eight ears, with a payoff of 2324 calories! Is oil a natural food?

Now, we know for sure that a certain amount of fatty acids is essential in the diet, particularly linoleic acid, which if too severely limited can produce dramatic effects.

There is argument over how much linoleic acid is actually needed, but we do know that the more saturated fat in the diet, the more linoleic acid is required. Top scientists are stating that on a 20 percent fat diet, 6 percent should be from linoleic acid. If one gets down to 10 percent fat, the amount of linoleic acid needed is considerably less. Let's assume that 6 percent linoleic acid is a good figure to shoot at. On a 2500-calorie diet, one could obtain this from 2.3 tablespoons of corn oil each day or one-third cup of walnuts or 0.4 cup of sunflower seeds. Since many other items in the natural diet (e.g., corn, wheat, rice, oats, millet, soybeans, chickpeas, and any nut or seed) contain linoleic acid, one wouldn't need this much from one source. It's easy to see that as our consumption of animal fat and other saturated fats decreases, our linoleic acid requirement more and more realistically can be met by eating natural foods in normal amounts. If the average American eliminated all the animal fat in his diet, instead of getting 40 percent of his calories from fat he would only get 20 percent from fat. If in addition he eliminated all hydrogenated fat products such as shortenings and margarines (and products containing them), he would get only 13 percent of his calories from fat. All this is without even changing the amount of oil consumed. Once oil consumption is reduced, linoleic acid requirements are simple to satisfy.

Does this mean you have to purge your pantry of all oils? Not necessarily. Oils are useful in preparing many foods, and forsaking them completely might result in too boring a diet for many people. Oils should, however, be considered a special food—one used sparingly and conservatively if superior health is to be realized. It is quite possible to live without oils and prepare excellent dishes, and a few recipes are included at the end of this chapter to give you an idea how easily oil can be eliminated.

The Polyunsaturate-Cholesterol Connection

Experiments were done some years back in which monkeys were fed a diet containing daily doses of corn oil, and their serum cholesterol levels were observed to lower significantly as a result.[7] It was concluded that the polyunsaturated fatty acids in the oil had the property of stripping cholesterol deposits off the artery linings, even if the diet was otherwise kept the same. This report kicked off the polyunsaturate fad of the 1970s, and oil and margarine manufacturers leaped on the opportunity to increase the sales of their products with this revelation. While it is true that polyunsaturated oils appear to lower serum cholesterol levels, the important question is where does the cholesterol and its associated fats go? The answer is that it is dumped into the gallbladder and into the bowel and is passed in large amounts, producing gallstones and possibly even colon cancer.[8] Hardly a profitable trade-off.

Now, if you are on a high fiber, low fat diet and are taking polyunsaturates to lower cholesterol, chances are these fats will be moved out of your digestive system fast enough to have little detrimental effect. But if you are on such a diet, you don't need polyunsaturates, since a low fat diet is usually a low cholesterol diet, and this in itself is sufficient to reduce cholesterol levels.

To sum up, continuing to eat the typical Western, high animal fat, high cholesterol diet and taking polyunsaturated oils to keep serum cholesterol readings down is merely trading one problem for another. The answer to safely reducing your cholesterol level is to stop or sharply limit your intake of cholesterol-rich, high saturated fat foods (i.e., animal foods). This will automatically get you on foods higher in fiber and thus solve a few other problems at the same time.

Recipes (Without Oil)

Mushroom Gravy[5]

½ lb. mushrooms, chopped
2 leeks, sliced
2¼ cups cold water
1 tsp. oregano

1 tsp. thyme
1 tbsp. salt-reduced tamari
3 tbsp. arrowroot

Sauté mushrooms and leeks in ¼ cup of water with the oregano and thyme for 10 minutes. Mix the arrowroot and tamari with 2 cups of cold water. Add to mushroom-leek mixture. Cook over low heat, stirring frequently, until it thickens (about 20 minutes). Makes about 2½ cups.

Chili[5]

¾ cup brown rice
2 cups dried kidney beans
7 cups water
2 onions, chopped
2 green peppers, chopped
6 cloves garlic, crushed

1 large can tomatoes (28 oz.) or 2 cups fresh chopped tomatoes plus
½ cup water
2 tsp. ground cumin
2¾ tsp. chili blend powder

Place beans, rice, and water in large pot. Cover and cook over low heat about 1 hour. Add remaining ingredients, breaking up canned tomatoes with a fork. Continue to cook, about 1½ hours longer (60 minutes covered, then 30 minutes uncovered). Serves 8.

Ratatouille[8]

½ eggplant, peeled and cut into chunks
1 cup sliced zucchini
1 green pepper, cut into chunks
1 large onion, cut into chunks
2 stalks celery, cut in diagonal slices (Chinese style)
2 shallots, finely chopped (optional)
1 clove garlic, minced
2 to 3 Tbsp. chopped fresh parsley
⅛ tsp. ground pepper
2 cups fresh tomatoes, cut into chunks, or diced canned tomatoes

Combine all the ingredients (except tomatoes) in a large pot or skillet. Cover and cook over low heat for about 20 minutes. Uncover and cook 15 minutes more over moderate heat, stirring to prevent scorching. Add tomatoes, heat through, but do not permit tomatoes to become mushy. Serve hot. Serves 8.

×Middle East Vegetable Stew[5]

6 potatoes, sliced
4 carrots, sliced
1 cauliflower, cut into flowers
1 broccoli, cut into pieces
2 onions, halved and sliced
2 zucchini, thickly sliced
2 cups water
4 cloves garlic, crushed
1 Tbsp. paprika
½ tsp. cumin

½ tsp. oregano
1 bay leaf
¼ tsp. dill
¼ tsp. marjoram
¼ tsp. thyme
pinch of each: tumeric, nutmeg, cinnamon, allspice, cloves, ginger, coriander, cardamom
2 Tbsp. cornstarch or arrowroot
2 Tbsp. water

Layer the vegetables in a large casserole dish in this order: potatoes, carrots, cauliflower, broccoli, onions and zucchini. Mix the water, garlic, and all herbs and spices. Pour over vegetables. Cover the casserole, place in a 350° oven for 1½ hours. When finished baking, remove from oven, drain juices into saucepan and heat. Make a paste of 2 Tbsp. cornstarch or arrowroot and 2 Tbsp. water. Add slowly to juice mixture, stir until thickened. Pour sauce over cooked vegetables and serve. Serve with brown rice or whole grain bread. Serves 8.

No Oil Potato Chips

Slice whole potatoes (with skins) as thin as possible and bake on a nonstick cookie sheet at 400° until crisp. Before baking you may add seasonings such as onion powder, garlic powder, spices, or tamari.

Fat Composition of Certain Common Foods (per Usual Serving)

Food	Amount	Calories	% Calories from fat	% Fat which is Saturated	% Fat which is Mono-unsaturated (Oleic Acid)	% Fat which is Polyunsaturated	Mg. Cholesterol
Flesh							
Beef	8 oz	802	83	48	44	8	214
Bacon	2 slices	143	49	32	47	21	70
Chicken, with skin	8 oz	565	43	30	42	28	184
Chicken, no skin	8 oz	447	28	28	46	26	179
Lamb	8 oz	423	66	56	36	8	222
Veal	8 oz	511	61	50	43	7	230
Cod	4 oz	89	3	NA*	NA	NA	57
Red Snapper	4 oz	106	8	NA	NA	NA	NA
White Sea Bass	4 oz	106	22	NA	NA	NA	NA
Salmon	4 oz	252	63	34	34	32	40
Tuna, in water	6.5 oz can	234	6	25	25	50	116
Shrimp	4 oz	103	8	NA	NA	NA	170
Lobster	4 oz	103	19	NA	NA	NA	103
Dairy							
Cheese, Cheddar	1 oz	113	72	56	34	10	28
Butter	1 tbsp	102	100	55	33	12	35
Cow's milk	1 cup	159	48	55	33	12	34
Goat's milk	1 cup	163	54	62	24	14	28
Eggs	1 large	82	64	31	43	26	251
Nuts							
Almonds	1 cup	849	82	8	67	25	0
Peanuts	1 cup	838	75	22	43	35	0
Oils							
Corn	1 tbsp	120	100	10	30	60	0
Cottonseed	1 tbsp	120	100	25	21	54	0
Olive	1 tbsp	120	100	11	44	45	0
Safflower	1 tbsp	120	100	8	15	77	0
Soy	1 tbsp	120	100	15	20	65	0

*NA = Not Available. Information on fish is scant, but with a few exceptions (e.g. salmon, trout) they are presumed to be fairly low in fat and that fat is predominantly polyunsaturated.

Fat Composition of Certain Common Foods (per 100 grams)

Food	Calories	% Calories from Fat	% Fat which is Saturated	% Fat which is Monounsaturated (Oleic Acid)	% Fat which is Polyunsaturated	Mg. Cholesterol
Flesh						
Beef	390	83	48	44	8	94
Bacon	665	49	32	47	21	77
Chicken, with skin	124	43	30	42	28	81
Chicken, no skin	107	28	28	46	26	79
Lamb	222	66	56	36	8	98
Veal	207	61	50	43	7	101
Cod	72	3	NA	NA	NA	50
Red Snapper	93	8	NA	NA	NA	NA
White Sea Bass	93	22	NA	NA	NA	NA
Salmon	221	63	34	34	32	35
Tuna, in water	127	6	25	25	50	63
Shrimp	91	8	NA	NA	NA	80
Lobster	91	19	NA	NA	NA	91
Dairy						
Cheese, Cheddar	398	72	56	34	10	99
Butter	716	100	55	33	12	61
Cow's milk	65	48	55	33	12	14
Goat's milk	67	54	62	24	14	
Eggs	163	64	31	43	26	548
Nuts						
Almonds	598	82	8	67	25	0
Peanuts	568	75	22	43	35	0
Oils						
Corn	884	100	10	30	60	0
Cottonseed	884	100	25	21	54	0
Olive	884	100	11	44	45	0
Safflower	884	100	8	15	77	0
Soy	884	100	15	20	65	0

Sources: U.S. Dept. of Agriculture Handbooks no. 8, no. 8-1, no. 456; also Feeley, R. M. et al., Cholesterol content of foods. *Journal of the American Dietetic Association* 61: 134, 1972.

Q. *What about eating on airplanes?*

A. Well, you can order food like brown rice and vegetables without butter if you call them a few days in advance. Personally, I distrust airline food so much I either don't eat at all or I brown bag it.

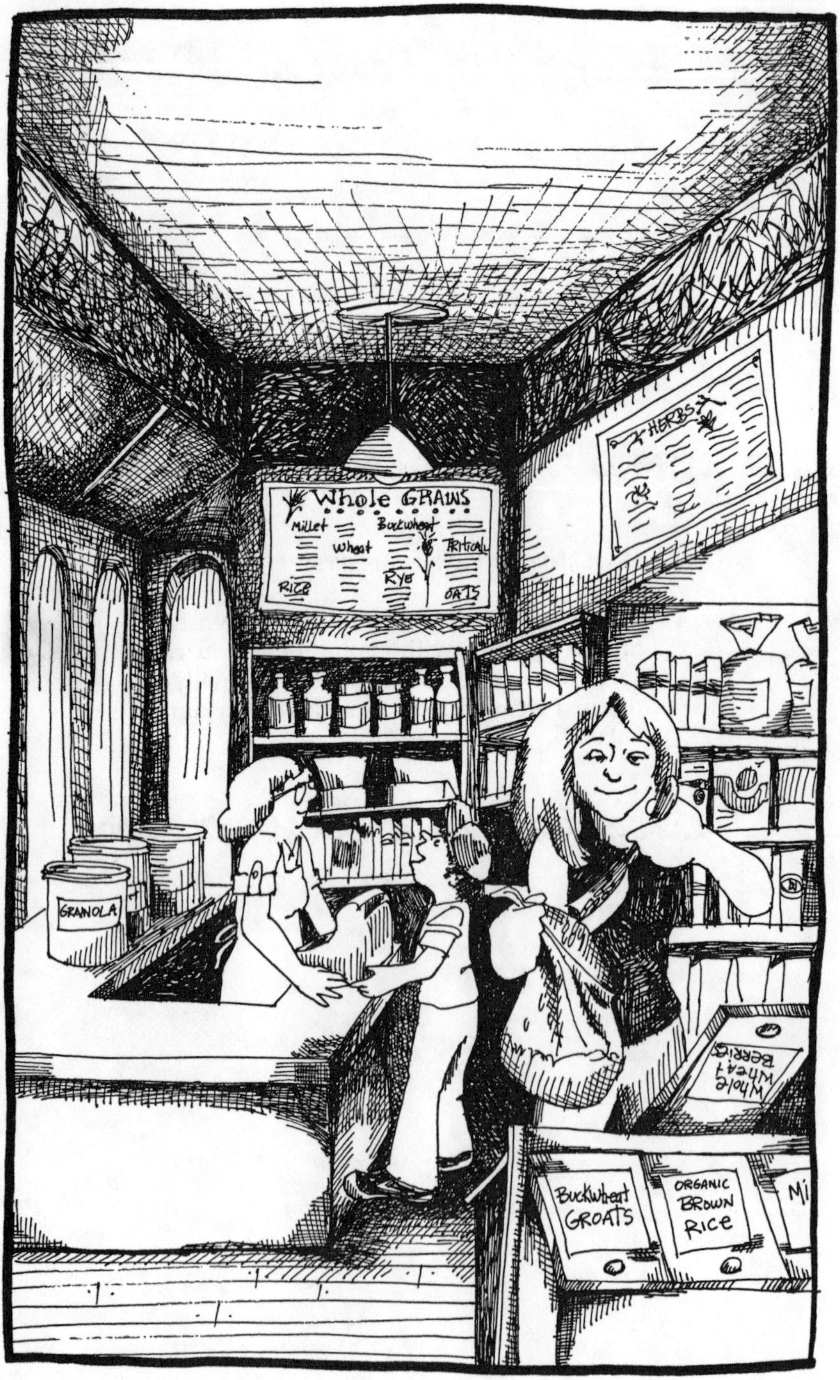
Whole GRAINS
Millet
Buckwheat
Wheat
Tritical
RICE
RYE
OATS
HERBS
GRANOLA
Whole Wheat Berries
Buckwheat GROATS
ORGANIC BROWN Rice

CHAPTER 6
Grains

As we enter the domain of real food, it is fitting that we start with grains, since they represent the world's most widely used staple food. They will be the centerpoint of any healthy, plant-based diet and your major source of protein and complex carbohydrates. With the exceptions of fruitarians, Eskimos, and the average Western teenager, most of us rely on grains directly or indirectly (grain is the major feed for cattle) for our energy. The majority of people in the West, of course, eat their grains in the form of bread or pasta, but the growing interest in both Eastern diet and natural foods in general is inducing more and more of us to eat grains in their whole unprocessed state. Steaming bowls of brown rice, millet, buckwheat, and even wheat and oats are slowly replacing the stacks of spongy white bread on the family dinner table. Homemade soups thick with barley, corn, and rye, fortified with beans and vegetables, are turning heads away from red and white cans of chicken noodle and cream of tomato soup.

Whenever grains are processed in any way that changes them from their whole, "as grown" state, something is sacrificed. The losses may be huge, as the table on the following page shows, comparing two major whole grains and their refined counterparts.

A casual glance reveals the destructive effects of the conversion to white rice or white flour. Even so-called enrichment does little to restore the many nutrients removed during refinement. Ironically enough, probably the single most important difference is not in vitamins and minerals at all, but in the nondigestible component, fiber. The lack of fiber so radically alters the digestive pattern of grain products that they behave more like sugars—rapidly absorbed energy sources which in the long run do more harm than good.

Comparison of Two Whole Grain Foods to Their Refined Enriched Counterparts with Respect to Certain Nutrients

Food per 100 grams	Energy calories	Protein grams	Fat grams	Total Carbohydrate grams	Fiber grams	Calcium milligrams	Phosphorus milligrams	Iron milligrams	Potassium milligrams	Thiamine (B₁) milligrams	Riboflavin (B₂) milligrams	Niacin milligrams
Whole Wheat	330	12.3	1.8	71.7	2.3	46	354	3.4	370	.52	.12	4.3
White Flour	365	11.8	1.1	74.7	.3	16	95	.9	95	.08	.06	1.0
Enriched White Flour	365	11.8	1.1	74.7	.3	16	95	2.9	95	.44	.26	3.5
Brown Rice	360	7.5	1.9	77.4	.9	32	221	1.6	214	.34	.05	4.7
White Rice	363	6.7	.4	80.4	.3	24	94	.8	92	.07	.03	1.6
Enriched White Rice	363	6.7	.4	80.4	.3	24	94	2.9	92	.44	.03*	3.5

*This figure is assumed to be the same as that for unenriched white rice until new data become available.
Source: U.S. Dept. of Agriculture Handbook no. 8.

The emphasis then should be on the use of whole, intact grains as much as possible. They may be used in soups and salads, as side dishes, or as main courses in an infinite variety of ways. Let's first look at the array of grains, both whole and processed, that you may encounter in a natural food store. Flours, rolled grains, and sprouted grains are mentioned here but discussed in more detail in later chapters.

Barley

When barley is harvested it has a tough pair of outer husks which is usually removed before it goes to market. "Whole" barley, therefore, is really partially hulled but still retains the *aleurone layer*, where the protein and a good proportion of the vitamins and minerals are found. Barley is excellent in soups and stews and barley flour may be used for breads, pies, and pancakes. Barley is also the major grain used for brewing beer.

Barley, Scotch

Here the aleurone layer has been removed, along with most of the nutrients and fiber. This is your standard white barley found in most commercial soups and baby foods, and is best avoided since it is not a whole food.

Buckwheat

Although buckwheat has nutritional characteristics similar to wheat, it is otherwise unrelated, belonging to a family of herbs and having been used as a grain since prehistoric times. In natural food stores, it will often be found in three different forms: whole buckwheat (sprouting buckwheat), raw buckwheat groats, and roasted buckwheat groats. Whole buckwheat has a tough black hull that is difficult to eat even after extensive cooking. It is generally cracked into a coarse meal, ground into flour, or used for sprouting (see Chapter 13). Raw groats make an excellent and easily prepared cereal, but don't expect them to taste like most of the grains you're accustomed to. They have a unique flavor and texture that sometimes reminds one more of beans than grain. Roasted groats have a nice nutty flavor, and since they are essentially cooked already may be added to quick cooking dishes like stir-fried vegies.

Corn

Although corn exists in a number of varieties, most of them are fed to cattle and hogs. The large yellow kernels seen in natural food stores are generally ground into cornmeal for baking and porridges, but they may be soaked and cooked into soups as well. Yellow corn is the most popular, the yellow pigment indicating a high vitamin A content, while the less often used white corn lacks this pigment and vitamin.

Millet

Often referred to as the "queen of the grains" and used extensively throughout much of the world, in America millet has been mostly relegated to the lowly position of birdseed. Lucky for the birds, since millet is a most nutritious grain, containing ample protein and an abundance of minerals, especially iron. Millet comes both hulled and unhulled, but recipes referring to "whole millet" mean the hulled variety, since it is most common. Although the unhulled seed has higher fiber content, ample fiber remains in the hulled variety. Hulled millet cooks up quickly and makes a delicious, highly digestible cereal. Unhulled millet may be ground into flour, cooked as a cereal grain, sprouted, or fed to your canary.

Oats

Most people are familiar with oats only in their rolled or steel cut form as breakfast cereals, but whole oats make a nice side dish or addition to soups. Tough outer husks, like those on barley, are removed prior to marketing, but all of the nutritional value is retained.

Popcorn

Its super hard outer hull makes it virtually inedible, but this very characteristic enables popcorn to pop. The high moisture content within the grain turns into steam as heat is applied, finally exploding the corn out of its casing. Although popcorn is a good source of fiber, some of its nutritional value is lost in popping. For most people, though, the real problem with popcorn is what they put on it. Gobs of melted butter and salt turn an otherwise harmless low calorie food into a vehicle for too much fat and too much sodium. Try using low-salt tamari in place of table salt, sprinkling on brewer's yeast for flavor, or just eating it plain.

Popcorn has traditionally been made by heating the kernels in hot smoking oil, but for those wishing to avoid oils and the potential rancidity of oils heated to high temperatures, electric corn poppers are now available which use only hot air to induce popping.

Rice, Brown

Like most grains, rice has a heavy outer husk which must be removed before eating. It is easier to accomplish this by "polishing," which also removes several other layers of the grain, than by a coarser method which would remove only the husk, leaving the nutrient-packed layers intact. This is one reason why white rice is less expensive than brown, another reason being that white rice has a far longer shelf life, since there is less in it to spoil.

Brown rice takes quite a bit longer to cook than white, but its nutritional benefits are well worth it, and once you've become accustomed to its coarser texture and nutty flavor you'll wonder why you ever liked white rice.

Natural food stores may sell brown rice in three lengths: short, medium, and long. Nutritional differences among the types are insignificant; the main factor is texture. Long grain will cook up dry and fluffy, while short grain will be soft and sticky. As you might expect, medium grain falls somewhere in between, but generally tends to behave more like long grain.

The uses of rice are many. It may be eaten hot or cold, whole or floured, as a main course, side dish, or dessert. It is a superior baby food when milled into a fine gruel and is highly digestible.

Rice, Sweet

The Japanese pound sweet rice into a sticky paste to make a dish called *mochi*. It is a superior, super short grain rice which is highly "glutinous," a term which refers to the stickiness of its starch molecules and should not be confused with "gluten," which is a type of protein found in wheat and certain other grains. If you couldn't care less about making *mochi*, you'll still find sweet rice appealing for its sticky quality and somewhat "sweet" taste.

Rice, White

Although white rice hardly qualifies as a natural food, since much of its nutritional value is discarded during polishing, many natural food stores stock it for two reasons. First, it represents a "transition" food for those who want to switch their families over to brown rice and find it easier to do so in gradual steps, by mixing varying proportions of brown and white rices until eventually the white rice disappears from the mixture. Second, the white rice sold by natural food stores should be free of a substance called asbestos. Most producers routinely coat their white rice with asbestos talc to discourage insect infestation. Warnings on packages may recommend that you "wash before using," but the problem is the stuff just doesn't wash off so easily. Laboratory tests have shown asbestos fibers still remaining after *nine* washings.[1]

At one time it was thought asbestos might be responsible for stomach cancer. However, some areas which do not use the talc-coated type of rice have a higher incidence of stomach cancer than those areas which do use it.[2] This does not mean that using talc-coated rice gives one some protection against stomach cancer, only that most cancers are probably related to multiple factors, both dietary and environmental. Nevertheless, with our current knowledge of the harmful effects of inhaled asbestos on the lungs, we might be well advised to wait until the issue has been settled before giving talc a clear bill of health.

Some producers, aware of the growing concern over asbestos, are choosing other potentially less hazardous coatings for their rice. If you're going to buy white rice at a supermarket, be sure it doesn't contain asbestos talc. That sold in natural food stores should be talc free, but don't take this for granted—ask! Brown rice will contain no coatings whatsoever.

Rice, Wild

This is one of those special treats you give yourself from time to time, and it is as delicious as it is expensive. Wild rice is not really a rice at all. It is an aquatic grass growing almost exclusively on Chippewa Indian land in the Great Lakes area, and also in China and Japan. Since very little is produced each year it can get quite costly, prices often ranging from $8 to $15 a pound in some areas. It is a natural whole grain, untreated and unpolished, with a rich hearty flavor that comes through even when only a small amount is mixed with ordinary brown rice, which is probably the best way to serve it considering its extraordinary cost.

Rye

Most often used as flour, rye can be a flavorful addition to soups and grain mixtures served as side dishes.

Sorghum

Occasionally you may find sorghum in a natural food store, but it is most often obtained wherever animal feed is sold. It is a staple grain of Africa, but rarely used on Western dinner tables.

Triticale

Loosely speaking, triticale is a cross between wheat and rye. It was developed for the purpose of creating a grain with the high protein and rising capacities of wheat and the sturdiness and adaptability of rye. Like rye, it is used primarily as flour.

Wheat, Durum

Anyone who has ever eaten pasta in any form has eaten flour made from durum wheat. The starch in durum wheat is far too hard to make edible bread, but that very quality makes it ideal for all manner of spaghetti, lasagne, vermicelli, and so forth, which has to stay together while being boiled, baked, fried, and steamed.

The whole grain pastas found in natural food stores are made from whole durum wheat flour, while the white flour pastas commonly sold in supermarkets and served in ordinary restaurants are made from a refined durum flour known as *semolina*, which lacks fiber and nutrients.

Wheat, Hard

Gluten is a protein found in wheat and the substance which causes baked goods made with wheat flour to rise when leavened with yeast or soda. Wheat designated as "hard" has a high proportion of gluten protein, usually 13 to 14 percent, and thus makes the best flour for bread baking. It is interesting that hard wheat tends to lower blood cholesterol whereas soft wheat does not.[3]

Wheat, Pastry

Lower in gluten, with a softer core, pastry wheat is excellent for baking cookies, cakes, and pastries, where lighter textures are desired. Pastry wheat flour works well with baking soda and powder but not so well with yeast.

Wheat, Soft

Same as pastry wheat.

Wheat, Spring

Spring wheat is planted in the spring and harvested in the fall.

Wheat, Winter

Winter wheat is planted in the fall, sprouts up before the snow arrives and is harvested in the spring. It has a larger yield than spring wheat but entails greater risk, since an early frost before snow comes can destroy the entire crop. Both spring and winter wheats have hard and soft varieties.

Any wheat can be used in its whole form as a staple food, although the hard wheats are generally preferred, due to their high protein value. Wheat "berries," as the whole grains are called, may be cooked up like rice and served as a side dish or added to soups. Try mixing about one part wheat berries to three parts brown rice and cooking them together. The wheat adds a pleasant crunchiness to a mushy rice.

Selection and Storage

A whole grain should be selected with the same critical eye one applies to the selection of an apple or a head of lettuce. Although grains have a far longer shelf life than fruits and vegetables they are nonetheless to be considered perishables. Unfortunately, the telltale signs of age and spoilage in grains are not nearly as obvious as a soft-skinned apple or wilted lettuce leaves. The primary concern is mold, which is a sign of either old grain or grain which has been improperly stored, allowing it to absorb too much moisture. Look carefully through your wheat or barley or rye for green or partially green grains. These are not immature but moldy grains. The exception to this rule is rice, where green grains are common. These *are* immature grains and should not concern you greatly.

What you want of course are the freshest grains possible, and mold is an obvious sign that you're not too close. But, just because a grain doesn't show mold today is no guarantee that it won't in a month or so, which means it's still pretty old. All in all, your best shot is to know your supplier, so to speak. What I mean by this is to shop around a bit until you find stores that specialize in the sale of commodities like grains and do a brisk business in them. This will assure you that the product turnover is fast and the products are therefore reasonably fresh. A store that specializes in vitamin pills but has a small token section of packaged rice, wheat, and various beans for the convenience of customers probably doesn't sell a great deal of this type of product. Since retailers are not apt to throw out stock unless it shows obvious signs of deterioration, you may be buying some fairly old grain in this store. It is wiser to buy your perishable foods from a place that sells more of them.

Another thing to keep an eye on is the store and storage temperature. Most grain has a good long shelf life if properly stored; say two years under ideal conditions, which means cool and dry. Temperatures above 70° will cause rapid deterioration of grain, and temperatures below 45° will guarantee long storage life. Check to see how your local merchant stores his grain. Is the shop hot during the day? Are grains exposed to sun continuously? Is the back-up inventory kept in a cooler?

Now, many natural food stores cannot afford the luxury of a walk-in refrigerator for storage, so don't be too hard on them.

However, the retailer with quality and freshness in mind can be sure to order his perishable products carefully so as not to have to store them for very long. No doubt his suppliers have properly controlled storage conditions.

Once you feel you've selected the best grain available, the second phase of storage is up to you. Obviously the ideal would be to keep all grains in the refrigerator, but this may not always be practical. If you're going to use your rice or wheat or whatever in a couple of weeks, a tightly sealed glass, metal, or plastic container will be fine—just keep it out of direct sunlight. If you plan to keep it for longer periods you'll have to think more about airtight containers and cool, dry places. Home storage is practical for up to a year or so under the right conditions, but stock should be used and replaced after that.

Walking Grains

If one morning you happen to glance over at your mason jar full of rice and see it moving, look a little closer, you're about to enter the Wonderful World of Weevils. Weevils are ant-sized insects that love natural foods, especially grains of all kinds. The eggs from which they hatch are microscopic and are usually present in all grains except those that have been specially treated for long-term storage, and even then there's no guarantee. So, if all grain contains weevil eggs, why aren't weevils overrunning all of our supplies? Mainly because they need the right conditions to hatch: sufficient time and high temperatures. Grain which is turned over quickly in shops and stored at low temperatures will rarely develop weevil infestation. It can happen, however, and it doesn't necessarily mean anything is wrong with the grain. In fact, you can be fairly confident that if the weevils are enjoying your wheat it hasn't spoiled.

So what to do with it? If you're the kind of person who is thoroughly horrified at the thought of eating anything that bugs have been playing in, you may as well throw it out and learn how to store your grains better. If you'd like to save the grain, however, there are some simple answers. The hatched weevils can be sifted out quite easily using an ordinary strainer, then the grain should be frozen for three days (72 hours), which will kill any you've missed. After this you can put it back on the shelf and forget it. If you were planning to use up the grain soon anyway, putting it in water is the easiest solution. The little buggers will float to the top and you can just scoop them off. Weevils are harmless little insects and nothing to be overly concerned about. Many hard-core natural food veterans just keep on eating, weevil and all, thankful for the extra protein.

Another natural food pest commonly encountered is the mealy moth. This little moth, with a wing span of only about ½ inch, has truly wreaked havoc in the natural food business in recent years. Mealy moths like to lay their eggs in grain and grain products (they especially love granola) and form cocoons out of which ultimately crawl tiny white worms which eventually become moths and lay their own eggs, repeating the cycle. Before long your jar of millet will be a virtual hotbed of life, full of cute little moths, fluttering about and bumping their little heads on the lid.

When it gets to this point you may as well let them have the victory and start over, but if you've got only one or two worms, just pick them out and freeze the grain for three days, which will destroy the eggs and save your food. You may as well learn how to save food whenever possible, since there might come a time in the not too distant future when you'll have no choice in the matter.

Your Grandmother Is Organic

It is virtually impossible to walk into a natural food store these days without seeing the word "organic" at least ten times in the first minute. Since the term is so commonly used and misused we should address the issue early on so that you can have a clear understanding of what it's all about.

Strictly speaking, something is organic if it contains carbon—which means that it is either living or has lived at one time; otherwise it is inorganic. By this rule a cucumber is certainly organic and so is your grandmother; but then so is gasoline, since it is derived from crude oil, which ultimately was made from the decomposed remains of plant life, dinosaurs, and probably some of your ancestors. Think about that the next time you start your car.

The word "organic" as it is used in the natural food industry is really short for "organically grown." A food is "organic" if it has been grown on completely natural soil without the use of chemical fertilizers. Some also include it to mean that the food has never been sprayed, dusted, or treated in any way with chemicals. Such a food is therefore "organic," in that no part of it contains substances like chemical pesticides, artificial colorings, waxes, etc.

So, what's so good about organic foods? From a strict scientific point of view we would have to admit that there is yet no evidence which demonstrates any nutritional advantage to organic farming. Many attempts have been made to show a difference between the nutritional qualities of organically grown and commercially grown foods, but none has satisfactorily demonstrated this to date. It is argued that every plant, from a carrot to a coconut tree, has a genetic code determining which nutrients it needs and in what amounts, which nutrients it will extract from the soil, and how it will grow. The carrot doesn't care whether those nutrients are from manure or some manufacturer, it either wants them or it doesn't. If a soil is genuinely *lacking* in an essential element, the carrot simply doesn't grow; or it grows in such an inferior way as to render it commercially useless. So, if a carrot seed becomes a grown up carrot it has done so because it has been provided with everything it required in order to grow. Iron is iron and zinc is zinc and nitrogen is nitrogen, whether it is "organic" or not.

This seems to be a cogent argument, but why am I not convinced? The nonscientific side of me keeps telling me there must be a flaw here somewhere. I refuse to admit that Man is capable of artificially duplicating a system as complex as that which grows food from the Earth. Perhaps we are being victimized by the limitations of our knowledge rather than humbled by it. Consider this if you will: the nutrient analyses upon which the value of organic growing methods are summarily dismissed are limited by: (1) the quality of our measurement instruments; and (2) the number of nutrients we are capable of testing for. Future developments may produce more sophisticated methods of analysis that will demonstrate differences previously undetectable, and our knowledge of food nutrients may broaden to include new substances that vary greatly between organic and commercial foods.

After all, we are aware that there are nutrients in food yet undiscovered, and these may be extremely important in maintaining optimum health. Most comparisons between organic and commercial foods only test for four or five key nutrients, yet even if all forty-odd known nutrients were shown to be in equal amounts, we still do not have any information on those unknown nutrients. Personally, as long as all the information is not yet in, I prefer to place my money on Nature.

On the other hand, when we come to the subject of chemical sprays, we have a little more definite information to base our feelings upon. The truly organic carrot is not sprayed with a pesticide as the commercial carrot most certainly is, and it is here that the real value of organic produce is shown. Pesticide sprays are potentially dangerous. No doubt about that.

Years ago, such a public fuss was made over the popular pesticide DDT that it was eventually banned for most commercial uses. In its place, however, have come many new agricultural chemicals, most of them far worse than DDT. Phosdrin, malathion, parathion, dieldrin, toxaphene, and a host of other deadly compounds are now being used liberally on practically everything we eat. Some of these are suspected carcinogens, and we are totally unknowledgeable about the long-term, cumulative effects of any of them. At Harvard Medical School it was shown that a *single exposure* to organophosphate pesticides can initiate dramatic changes in human brain activity lasting for more than a year. A study at the National Cancer Institute has shown toxaphene, a pesticide used on many vegetables and grains, to cause liver cancer in mice.

One of the criticisms often heard from laymen about findings that this chemical and that chemical cause cancer in laboratory animals is that the animals are given doses so large that people would have to take in impossible amounts to get the same effect. This is not clear thinking at all. These chemicals are cumulative in the human system, and there is also evidence that they act synergistically, that is, many different chemicals which we ingest may act together to produce an amplified effect. Although you don't drink a gallon of substance X in one month, you may consume that over a thirty- or forty-year period. Besides, there is no clear understanding of just how much or how little of some substances may be carcinogenic. Cancer is a time bomb. Perhaps as little as a single molecule of a chemical may manifest its results twenty-five years later. But, if the body is nourished properly, and the immune system is functioning at its optimum, I believe most of these foreign invaders can be dealt with successfully.

Organic Grains

Most natural food stores carry a certain amount of organically grown grains. Some stock only organic grains and others offer a choice. While some grains are not heavily sprayed, a few, like rice in particular, are. If you're at all concerned about pesticides, it may be worth the extra investment to purchase organic rice.

Two questions that always arise are (1) How do I know it's organic? and (2) Why is it so much more expensive?

There is no guaranteed method of determining the *organicness* of a food product simply by visual inspection. Sometimes the organic food looks better, sometimes worse. The only real assurance you have lies in the integrity of your dealer. Most proprietors of natural food stores have a high level of consciousness about this sort of thing and will be honest. No doubt there are unscrupulous people in this as in every business, and as in all things a certain amount of faith is required. You can, of course, always question your merchant about the source of his organic grains. Arrowhead Mills (Deaf Smith), Chico-San, Erewhon, and Lundberg are good names to remember since they are all bona fide and reputable distributors of organically grown grains. If your dealer buys from these people, he's buying quality organic stuff, and he should be proud to tell you so. Of course, if you don't mind being a pest, you can ask him to show you the sack the grains come in. He'll no doubt grumble a bit but should understand your right to know.

When crops are grown organically they are more susceptible to damage from insects and rodents. Although there are certain natural, nonchemical ways to reduce the amount of destruction pests may cause, a certain level has to be tolerated. Pests have to eat too, after all, and the natural balance of things must be respected if we are to live in harmony with the Earth. Since the organic farmer loses a larger percentage of his crop to pests, his saleable crop will be smaller, yet his investment in time and land the same, and his family has to eat too. Obviously, if he is to continue as a farmer he is going to have to get a higher price for his product, and hope that the consumer is willing to pay the premium.

The Organic Rip-off

Since the term "organic" still has no legal definition, advertisers are free to use it however and whenever they please. And as the big-time food processors realize more and more that the public's concern over wholesome, additive-free foods is not just a passing fad, terms like "natural" and "organic" will be thrown around indiscriminantly whenever a profit can be made. All sorts of products are now popping up with "natural" and "organic" plastered all over them, when in fact they are just the same old stuff. How can a cereal claim to be 100 percent natural when over 20 percent of it is refined white sugar? Simple—without a legal definition, sugar may be considered natural, since after all it was derived from sugar cane or sugar beets, even though every bit of nutrition (except calories) has been taken out of it.

At this writing the Federal Trade Commission has a recommendation before it which would limit the use of these terms according to strict definitions. Foods claimed to be organic would have to be grown only with certain types of fertilizers and without the application of synthetic chemicals. If the FTC adopts these recommendations, we will have taken an important step toward enforced truth in advertising.

Preparation

Although most people first come in contact with grains in baked goods, granola, oatmeal, cracked wheat cereal, and other fragmented forms, preparing and eating them in their whole, natural state is by far the best method—their full nutritional benefits are realized and the chances of rancidity minimized.

Basic preparation of grains is simple. Begin by washing thoroughly using a strainer or by soaking several times for a few minutes and pouring off the soak water. Grains are raw agricultural products and will always contain a little dirt. The following table shows the ratio of grains to water for some you'll be using. Just bring the water to a boil, add grains, bring to a boil again, turn the heat low and let simmer gently in a covered pot for the duration of the cooking time or until all the water has been absorbed.

Some stoics can sit down to a big plate of plain brown rice and appear to be enjoying themselves, but for most of us some kind of seasoning is necessary to offset the basic blandness of grain. Cooking it up with lots of butter and salt may not be the healthiest approach. We all might do well to learn to appreciate the subtle flavors of the multitude of fine herbs and spices available

How to Cook Grains

Grain (1 cup)	Water	Time*	Yield
Brown Rice	2 cups	45 min.	3 cups
Barley	3 cups	60 min.	3½ cups
Buckwheat, raw groats	2 cups	20 min.	3 cups
Millet, unhulled	3 cups	45 min.	3½ cups
Millet, hulled	2 cups	20 min.	3 cups
Wheat, hard	3 cups	60 min.	3½ cups

*If you mix various grains together, cook according to the *whole* grain with the shortest cooking time, the longer cooking grains will just be crunchier. This does not apply when *hulled* grains like millet or buckwheat are used in a mixture.

to us. Here are a few suggestions for spicing up your rice or other grains.

Sweet flavor—cinnamon, allspice, cloves
Italian flavor—basil, oregano, parsley, spearmint, garlic, onions, bell pepper
Indonesian flavor—ginger, coriander, cumin
Indian flavor—curry powder
South American flavor—chili blend powder
My favorite—tarragon, dill weed, spearmint

Spices are best added a few minutes before the grain is finished cooking so their flavors will permeate the food yet not be destroyed by overheating. Naturally, amounts will vary according to taste, but as a rule of thumb figure on using two teaspoons of combined spices for each cup of raw rice if the spices are of the leafy type (like basil, oregano, tarragon, etc.), and half that amount if powdered spices are used (cinnamon, curry, cumin).

Recipes

Barley-Mushroom Casserole[3]

2 onions, chopped
½ lb. mushrooms, chopped
2½ cups boiling water
1 cup barley

½ tsp. thyme
¼ tsp. garlic powder
½ Tbsp. salt-reduced tamari

Sauté onions in ¼ cup water for 10 minutes, add mushrooms and sauté 5 minutes longer. Then add barley to the pot and stir and cook for 5 minutes more. Remove from heat. Add 2½ cups boiling water. Mix well. Add seasonings. Pour into casserole dish, cover, and bake in a 350° oven for about 1¼ hours. Serves 6–8.

Italian Buckwheat Rolls

1 cup raw buckwheat groats
2 cups water
8 large leaves green cabbage
1 large onion, chopped
3 cloves garlic, minced
1 Tbsp. olive oil
1 Tbsp. salt-reduced tamari
1 tsp. oregano
1 tsp. tarragon
1 tsp. dill weed
½ cup grated cheese (optional)
1 cup tomato sauce

Sauté onions and garlic in oil until soft. Add water, buckwheat, tamari, spices. Bring to a boil, reduce heat to low and simmer about 20 minutes or until all the water is absorbed. Steam cabbage leaves until soft enough to roll, roll buckwheat mixture up in them and place in casserole dish, seam side down. Pour tomato sauce over top and sprinkle with cheese, if desired. Bake at 350° for 30 minutes. Serves 2–3.

Gourmet Rice

2 cups long-grain brown rice
½ cup wild rice
½ cup soft wheat berries (pastry wheat)
4½ cups water
2 onions, chopped
2 to 4 cloves garlic
1 Tbsp. tarragon
1 Tbsp. spearmint (optional)
1 Tbsp. dill weed (optional)
tamari to taste

Sauté onion and garlic in tamari and a little water in a large pot. When soft, add rices, wheat, and water and bring to a boil. Lower heat and simmer covered for 45–50 minutes or until all water is absorbed. Add spices, mix well, and let sit for 15 minutes covered, off heat. Serves 3–4 as a main dish along with a salad or steamed vegies.

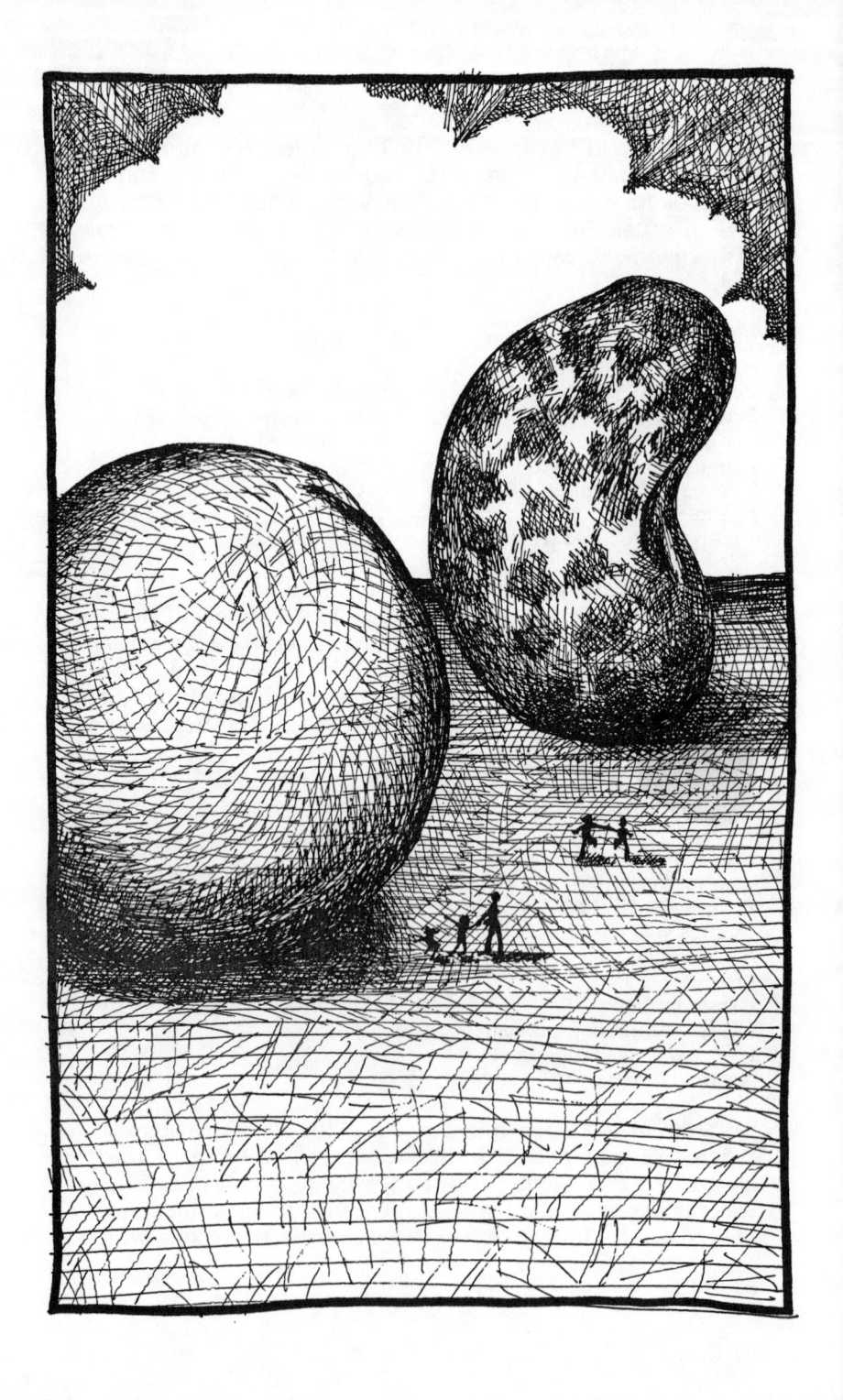

CHAPTER 7
Beans and Peas

Collectively, beans and peas, including peanuts, are referred to as *legumes* in the U.S., but more often as *pulses* in other countries. Some are ground into flour or cracked into grits, but for the most part they are used as a whole food. Certainly nothing comparable to the milling of wheat into white flour or the polishing of brown rice occurs to beans, with the exception of soy milk powder and textured soy protein, so they fit neatly into our definition of natural foods.

The low social status of beans as a staple food stems from a combination of poor public image and bad press. Beans are so often associated with poverty and peasant diets that they have slowly been excluded from the dinner tables of increasingly affluent societies. As we get richer, or at least think we're getting richer, we choose to eat the foods of the rich. Unfortunately, along with the foods of the rich go the diseases of the rich, while the lowly bean-eating peasants just keep on going, unable to share in the pleasures of diabetes, cancer, and heart disease.

And of course there's the problem of flatulence, or intestinal gas, a phenomenon that has been the curse of mankind since the invention of the crowded elevator. "Did you eat beans last night for dinner?" comes the sly question, as the perpetrator attempts to disguise himself as a potted plant. True, beans often produce some flatulence due to a certain amount of nondigestible carbohydrate being acted upon by colonic bacteria, and although I have heard of many techniques for cooking "gas-less" beans, none seems to work for everybody. What does seem to work is simple meals. If you eat a staple dinner of rice, beans, and vegetables, you are likely to have only minor flatulence, while adding foods like fruits and dairy products will give you enough gas to open a Mobil station.

As a food, beans are a lot more versatile than they are normally given credit for. The traditional image is an unappetizing pile of beans on a bare plate, perhaps accompanied by an equally boring mound of rice or corn. Sounds great if you happen to be involved in long-term guerilla warfare, but for most of us it's a bit too basic. Beans make good soups, of course, but also great sandwich spreads, dips, salad dressings, and meat replacers or extenders in all sorts of loaves and casseroles. Many beans may also be ground into flour for use in baking breads.

Nutritionally, beans have some pros and cons. They are a little too high in protein and should probably be used in the diet no more than a few times a week, especially soybeans and lentils. Their fat content is acceptable, with the exception of soybeans, which derive 40 percent of their calories from fat. The best thing about beans is their fiber, which appears to be one of the best known substances for lowering blood cholesterol.[1] Here are some of the beans and peas commonly available in natural food stores.

Azuki Beans (Aduki, Adzuki, Asuki)

Common to Japanese cooking, azukis are small brownish-purple beans with a black spot. They are excellent when sprouted, tasting much like fresh peas.

Black Beans

Sometimes called *turtle beans*, black beans are a South American staple with a rich full flavor. Their unusual color, unusual at least for a natural food, makes them an interesting addition to the table. They are most often used in simple dishes, spiced up and served with rice, or as black bean soup.

Blackeyed Peas

It seems almost impossible to say "blackeyed peas" without affecting a southern drawl, so strong is their association with the South. Also known as *cowpeas*, these little spotted peas are generally cooked in simple ways as soups or side dishes, and may be ground into flour for baked goods.

√ *Garbanzo Beans*

Also known as *chickpeas*, garbanzos are common in dishes of Middle Eastern origin, but are also used in some South American and Mediterranean cooking. Fairly obscure in the West until recently, garbanzos are now gaining popularity due to a new interest in Middle Eastern foods. Dishes such as *hummous* (a garbanzo dip) and *falafel* (sort of a meatball made from beans) are becoming widely known. Garbanzo flour is also getting pretty popular, and is useful especially for those with wheat-related allergies.

√ *Kidney beans*

Along with split peas and navy beans, kidneys are among the beans most commonly used in America. They were always the funny shaped beans in Grandma's soup, and as life went on and there was no more Grandma's soup and you had to cope with a can of chili for dinner, there they were again. Kidneys are what one might call a "hearty" bean. They are quite flavorful and "meaty" and may be used in a variety of cooked dishes and as cold salad beans.

√ *Lentils*

Most people have never seen a whole lentil, which is a pair of flat peas inside a common husk. What we see is the separated peas after the husk is removed. They are still whole beans, however, and husking destroys no nutrients. Lentils are a staple food in India, where they are called *dhal*, but are widely used throughout Europe and the U.S. as well. The natural foods movement has given lentils a major popularity boost, and no natural foods cookbook seems to lack recipes for lentil soup, lentil loaf, and lentil burgers. Lentils are readily available, moderately priced, tasty, versatile, and easy to prepare. Because they are so flat and thin, they are one of the few beans that need not be soaked overnight before cooking, taking one of the major hassles out of beans—planning ahead. Their relatively high protein content makes them a natural for vegetarians bored with soybeans; and they are the least likely to cause flatulence.

√ *Mung Beans (Mungo)*

Somewhere out there, there may be someone who has never eaten in a Chinese restaurant, but I've never met him. Unless you are him, you've undoubtedly eaten mung beans, for it is from this tiny green bean that the world famous Chinese bean sprout emerges. The bean itself is occasionally used whole in Chinese cookery, but it is almost always the sprout that prevails. As you will find in Chapter 13, sprouting is a simple and economical way to produce tasty and highly nutritious vegetables at home.

Peanuts

Most of us think of peanuts as nuts, but in fact they are a type of pea belonging to the legume family. Nutritionally, however, they do seem closer to nuts, especially with regard to their high protein, high oil, and high calorie contents.

Peanuts may be eaten raw or roasted, in the shell or shelled. Since the shell provides natural protection against spoilage, the ideal way to eat peanuts, and all nuts for that matter, is by shelling them yourself.

Roasted peanuts tend to spoil far more quickly than raw, so keep a close watch on them. If the oils in peanuts go rancid, they will have a "musty" odor and will produce a burning sensation in the back of your throat a few moments after you've eaten them.

The two most common varieties of peanuts are *Spanish* and *Virginia*. The raw version of the Spanish peanut is often called a *redskin,* due to the dark red skin left on the outside. This skin has a slightly bitter taste that some people find not to their liking. It has no particular nutritional value, and may contain toxins, although this is nothing to be seriously concerned about unless your diet is based heavily on peanut skins. When the skins are removed and the peanuts roasted, you've got the raw material for peanut butter, the Spanish being preferred since they are smaller, softer, and easier to grind smooth. If you want to make raw peanut butter, you'll probably have to add some oil, since raw peanuts produce a powder or powdery paste when ground. Roasting liquifies the oils and heightens the taste.

Virginia peanuts may be found in at least six different forms: raw in the shell, roasted in the shell, raw redskins, roasted redskins, raw blanched, and roasted blanched. *Blanching* is a method of removing the skin by dropping the peanuts in boiling water for a few seconds, a process which does not depreciate the nutritional value to any great degree.

Most natural food stores offer unsalted peanuts, while supermarket brands are almost inevitably salted. If reducing the amount of sodium in your diet is a concern, and it should be, take care with salted peanuts. You can take in an awful lot of salt quickly this way. And don't assume that peanuts still in the shell are necessarily unsalted, since they've apparently found a way to get salt inside the shell.

Peanuts are considered strictly as munchies by most people, but they are quite versatile in all sorts of recipes. Lots of exotic Indonesian and African dishes are based on peanuts, and you can use them in soups, sauces, casseroles, and much more. Even peanut flour can be used in baked goods.

Peas, Green

Green peas, in dried form, are found in both whole and split versions. Whole green peas are the ones that always seem to be hanging out with carrots, but by themselves may be added to soups or sprouted into a tasty vegetable.

Only someone with a deprived childhood has not had a hot bowl of split pea soup on a cold winter's day. The standard split pea soup, of course, usually had a big ham hock floating around in it, but meatless recipes abound and you'll never miss the pig. Split peas, like lentils, have the advantage of cooking in a relatively short time, and overnight soaking is not mandatory, although it will reduce cooking time and save energy.

Split peas are found in green and yellow varieties and both are used in pretty much the same way. I've yet to find a nutrient analysis of yellow peas, so I can't say if one is better than the other, but since peas and beans are primarily protein and carbohydrate, any difference probably isn't important.

Since split peas have had their outer hull removed, they have lost most of their fiber. However, if they are used in a diet consisting largely of whole grains and vegetables, this lack of fiber is unimportant.

Pinto Beans

Now, if you live in California or any part of the Southwest, pinto beans are an old friend. Only a genius could prepare a full on Mexican dinner without pintos. The famous refried beans, without which no Mexican restaurant could exist, are pintos which have been cooked, mashed into a paste, and briefly "fried" in some kind of fat, along with nice things like onions, garlic, and spices. The fat used is most often lard, an animal fat, and if you want to avoid that, you'd best stay out of Mexican restaurants.

Soybeans (Soya Beans)

Volumes have been written about the soybean, the most widely known and used bean in the world. Staggering amounts are grown throughout the midwestern United States, mostly to feed livestock being grown for eventual slaughter. It has been calculated that 16 pounds of protein in the form of soybeans and other plant products must be fed to cattle to produce one pound of protein in the form of meat. This is obviously a flagrant waste of food and energy, since the soybeans could provide protein directly to humans, and the excess food would feed the world.

Because soybeans are so abundant they have become the Great White Hope of those who envision a meatless world. Their high protein and oil content, along with remarkable versatility, make them the perfect meat substitute, although for our purposes they are a bit too high in both these components. Soybeans have been prepared in a mind-boggling array of "mock" foods for vegetarians wanting a substitute for meat in their diets, or others who simply choose to cut back on meat consumption for health or economic reasons (see Chapter 17). For those wishing to eliminate dairy products from their diets, there seems to be a soy food for every occasion: soymilk, soy cheese, soy butter, soy egg replacer—yes, even soy ice cream.

Cooked by themselves, soybeans are exceptionally bland, but it is this very "neutral" characteristic which enables soy to change its character with the addition of herbs, spices, and so forth. As you read on, the amazing versatility of soybeans will become obvious to you; you find them popping up in the most unlikely places. Incidently, fresh soybeans may be found occasionally in markets, but do not eat them raw for they contain toxins which inhibit growth and digestion.[2]

Winged Beans

Winged beans are not now available in many places, but I anticipate they will be quite popular in the near future and thought you might want to become acquainted early. The winged bean is being billed as the "soybean of the tropics," since it is at least as nutritious as soy but can grow in places where the soybean cannot, especially in the hot, humid areas of the world, which house most of our planet's poor and often undernourished people.

The most impressive aspect of the winged bean is that the bean itself is only one of the plant's six edible parts. The pods, leaves, tendrils, flowers, and root are each remarkable vegetables in their own right. The potato-sized root is practically the entire diet of Papua New Guinea tribesman, a group known throughout the world for superior health and freedom from degenerative disease.

And More . . .

Lots of other beans will be found in recipes and in your local stores—great northerns, whites, navy beans, pink beans, red beans, fava beans, and so on. Most of these are similar and present no special features or problems. Any bean may be sprouted or cooked, and I leave it to you to find your favorites.

Selection and Storage

Beans do not present nearly as many problems as grains when it comes to freshness. Dried beans rarely if ever go rancid (peanuts being the one important exception), and mold is not a problem unless they get wet and are stored in such a way that they cannot dry out easily. Beans are good for at least two years stored under moderate temperatures, and in my experience they do not seem especially popular with weevils and mealy moths, although I have occasionally found lentils to be infested. However, I have seen some pretty faded looking beans in supermarkets and health food stores, and as in the case of grains you are wiser to buy your beans from a dealer who moves a lot of them in and out of his store.

You will probably have to wrestle with the organic/commercial decision with some beans, as many stores offer both. Beans are one agricultural crop that is not sprayed heavily since they don't have much of a pest problem. But, they are sprayed sometimes and if this is important to you, by all means seek out organically grown beans. If the price difference between the organic and commercial is great, and it shouldn't be, this may be one area where the budget-minded can cut corners and go with the cheaper commercially grown product.

Preparation

Many good distributors wash and dry grain before bagging it and shipping it off, but beans are rarely cleaned and it is always necessary to give them a thorough rinsing. You may also want to sort through them a bit, picking out any stones or twigs.

With the exception of lentils and split peas, beans should be soaked overnight to soften them and thus greatly reduce cooking time. If you forget to soak them, use this shortcut: cover beans with water and bring to a boil, turn off the heat and let them rest for one hour. This accomplishes pretty much the same thing as overnight soaking.

Cook beans basically the same as grains. Just add water, bring to a boil, turn the heat to low and simmer in a covered pot until they are tender, adding more water as needed. The following table shows some measurements and cooking times.

How to Cook Beans (Pre-soaked)

Beans (1 cup)	*Water*	*Time*	*Yield*
Lentil and Split Peas*	3 cups	1 hr.	2 cups
Pinto Beans	3 cups	2½ hrs.	2 cups
Red Beans	3 cups	3 hrs.	2 cups
White Beans	3 cups	1½–2 hrs.	2 cups
Garbanzos	4 cups	3 hrs.	2 cups
Blackeyed Peas	3 cups	1 hr.	2 cups
Black Beans	4 cups	1½ hrs.	2 cups
Soybeans	3 cups	3 hrs.	2 cups

*Do not need pre-soaking.

Recipes

x Black Beans and Rice

Beans
2 cups black beans
8 cups water
1 large onion, chopped
3 cloves garlic, chopped
2 green bell peppers, chopped
2 Tbsp. chili blend powder
1 Tbsp. tamari

Rice
2 cups brown rice
4 cups water
salt, if desired

Bring rice and water to boil. Lower heat, simmer covered 45–50 minutes.

Soak beans overnight. Cook all ingredients together 1½ hours.

Spoon beans over rice and serve with salad. Serves 4.

Simple Hummous

2 cups cooked garbanzo beans
3 oz. tahini
1 tsp. seasalt
1 tsp. garlic powder

Puree garbanzos in juicer or food processor (blender will work, but not quite as well). Mix in all other ingredients. Serve as a dip or as sandwich spread. Also makes a good base for salad dressings.

Split Pea Chowder[7]

6 cups water
½ cup brown rice
2 cups split peas
2 tsp. salt
1 cup sautéed onions
½ cup finely diced carrots
½ cup finely diced celery
½ tsp. sweet basil

Add rice to rapidly boiling water in large kettle. Cover. Bring to full boil and let cook 30 minutes. Add peas and cook 30 minutes more. Add salt, sautéed onions, carrots, and celery and let cook 10–15 minutes. Add basil, test, and season to taste. Serve over slices of whole wheat bread.

✓ Refried Beans

6 cups water
2 cups pinto beans
1 onion, chopped
3 cloves garlic, chopped

1 tsp. salt
2 tsp. cumin, ground
2 Tbsp. salt-reduced tamari

Soak pintos overnight, add salt, bring to a boil and simmer 2 hours. Pour off bean water into separate container. In a saucepan, sauté the onions and garlic in some of the bean water. Add this back into the beans along with cumin and tamari. Mash with potato masher or wire whisks until consistency of mashed potatoes, adding bean water as needed, and cook 15 more minutes on low heat, stirring frequently. Serve with rice, on chapattis or tortillas, or use as sandwich spread, hot or cold.

Sweet and Sour Lentil Soup

4 cups water
2 cups lentils
1 28 oz. can tomato puree
   or equal amount of pureed
   fresh tomatoes)
1 onion, chopped
2 carrots, sliced
⅓ cup apple cider vinegar

⅛ cup honey
2 bay leaves
1 Tbsp. garlic powder
1 Tbsp. basil
1 Tbsp. oregano
2 vegetable bouillon cubes

Combine all ingredients except vegetables. Bring to a boil, then simmer on low heat for 1 hour. Add vegetables and cook 15 minutes more. Serves 8.

Peanuts and Bulgur

1 cup bulgur
1¾ cups water
1 cup celery, chopped
1 cup onions, chopped
½ cup shelled roasted peanuts

1 Tbsp. tarragon
½ tsp. garlic powder
¼ tsp. ginger, ground
2 Tbps. salt-reduced tamari

Combine bulgur, water, celery, and onions and bring to a boil. Turn off heat, add remaining ingredients and let sit covered for 20 minutes. Serves 2.

Q. *My wife and I both work and can't wait hours for beans and rice to cook for dinner. Is there any fast way to prepare these foods?*

A. As far as rice and beans go, one solution is to make up large amounts once a week and refrigerate or freeze them in portions for your workdays. Rice and other grains will keep fine in the refrigerator for a week, and you can just steam them in a little water to heat them up. Beans seem to last forever in the refrigerator and will freeze very well, as will soups.

Another solution is a slow-cooker that will cook all day, or a stove with a timer you can pre-set to turn on at a certain time. Beside this, there are lots of whole foods which may be prepared in 30 minutes or less. Buckwheat, millet, bulgur wheat, whole wheat pasta, sliced potatoes, etc. Or how about just a big salad and whole wheat bread?

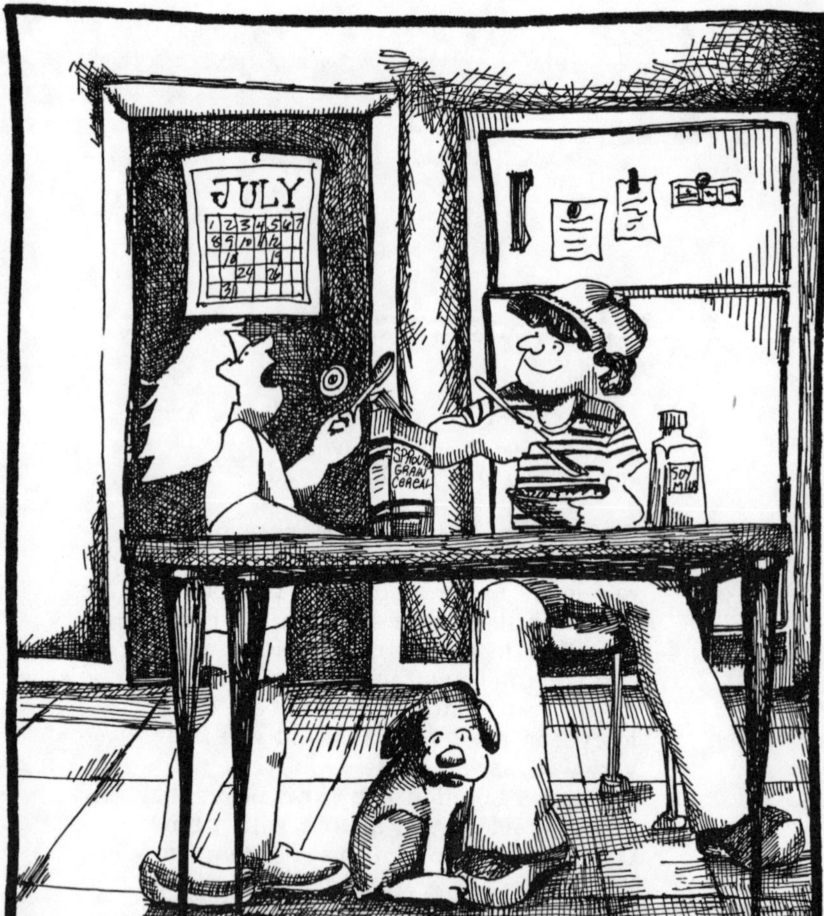
JULY
GRAIN
CEREAL
SUGAR
CRUNCHIES

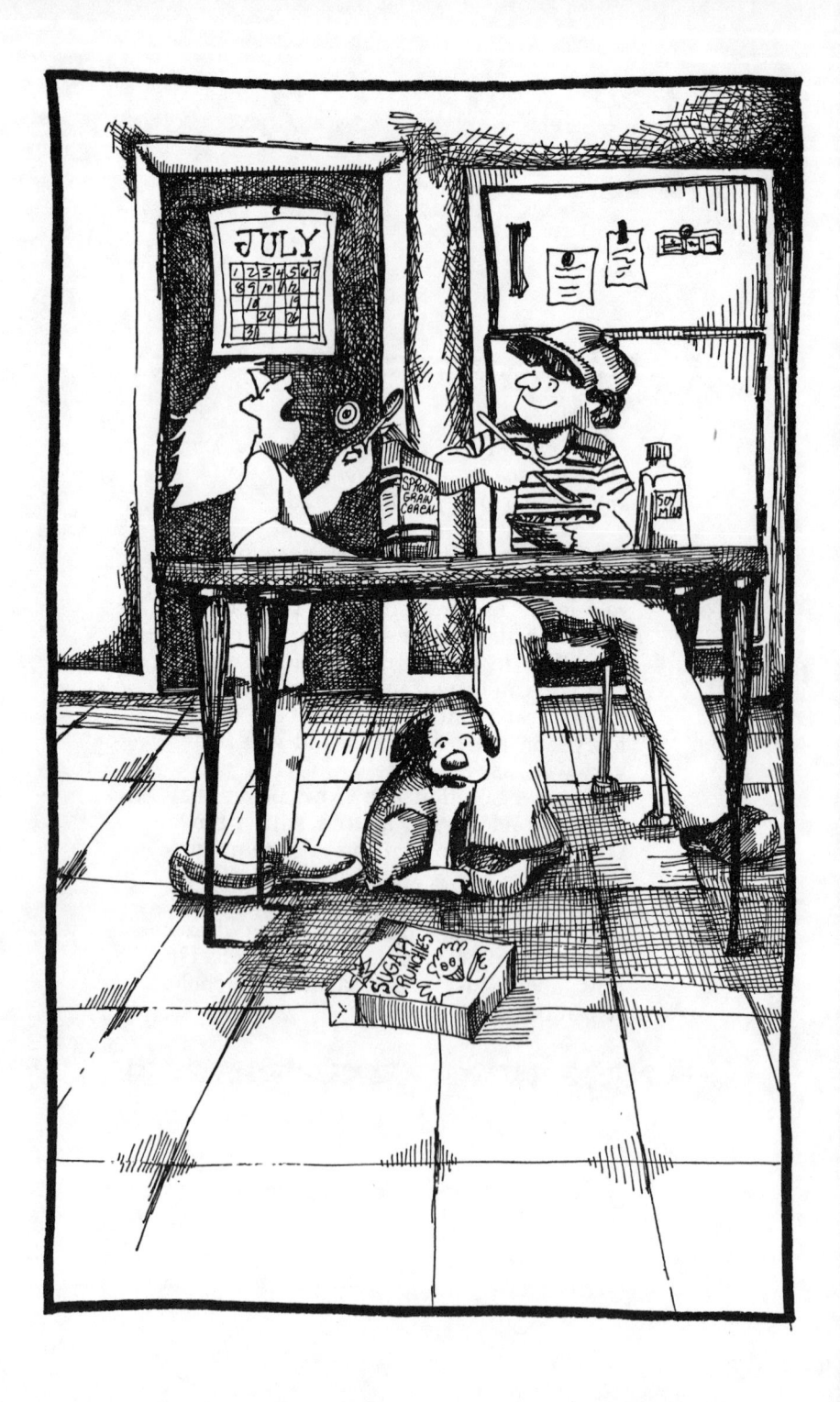

CHAPTER 8
Breakfast Cereals

Technically speaking, "cereals" is another way of saying "grains," and the terms are used interchangeably in world food markets. However, we use "cereal" here for that class of partially processed grains that people who eat natural foods normally associate with breakfast, although as we shall see, cereals have expanded their influence to snacks, lunch, and dinner.

Cereal grains are processed into at least six forms, each differing in texture, convenience of preparation, and nutritional value. The following list is in descending order of "wholeness."

Hulled Whole Cereals

This refers mainly to hulled buckwheat and hulled millet, both of which may be classified as cereals since they cook in about 20 minutes as compared to 45 minutes or more for whole grains. The "processing" here, the removal of the outer husk, does not significantly alter the nutritional value of the grain.

Grits

Here the whole grain is cracked into pieces, a process which greatly reduces cooking time since more surfaces are directly exposed to heat. Some loss of nutrients occurs when the inner layers of grain are subjected to air and light. Examples are cracked wheat, corn grits, barley grits, and soy grits. Grits generally cook in 15 to 20 minutes.

Shredded Cereals

These are the closest you'll get to "wholeness" in a cereal manufactured by the giant mills. Shredded wheat is made from the whole grain and so includes the germ and bran, and these cereals often are not loaded with sugar. Needless to say, some nutrient loss occurs during the shredding and toasting, but it is not great.

Flakes

The flaking process differs from grain to grain due to individual characteristics. In general the grain is heated, usually by steaming, rolled flat, and dried. In this way we can produce wheat flakes, rye flakes, barley flakes, triticale flakes, soy flakes, and oat flakes. These are also often referred to as rolled wheat, rolled rye, and rolled oats, commonly made into oatmeal.

Heating and flattening diminishes nutrients, but flakes remain good solid nutritious foods, certainly as compared to some breakfast cereals offered in most supermarkets.

Creams

Cream cereals are simply whole grain flour mixed with water and cooked—cream of wheat, cream of rye, cream of anything. Rice cream is an excellent cereal for infants owing to the easy digestibility of rice. Nutritionally, creams range from excellent, if made from freshly ground, 100 percent whole grain flour, to poor, if made from processed flour that has been sitting around in a box for six months.

Puffed Cereals

Puffed cereals are produced by heating moist grains and then suddenly dropping the pressure in the cooking unit. This causes steam to expand rapidly, exploding the grains. Puffed cereals have a pleasant texture but nutritional losses are greater than in most types of cereal. El Molino is one reputable company producing whole grain puffed cereals in four varieties: wheat, corn, rice, and millet.

Supermarket versions are mixtures of various grains, flours, dyes, sugars, flavorings, vitamins, salt, and preservatives rather than straight whole grains.

Here are several cereals you may encounter in your local natural food store:

Bran

This generally refers to wheat bran although *rice bran* is often available too. Wheat bran may be called *Miller's bran* as well, or simply *unprocessed bran*. Bran is the outside layer of the wheat berry, which is removed when whole wheat is processed into white flour. Although it contains a good many nutrients, some are not available to the human body since we are not able to digest bran completely. This very fact, however, makes it such a valuable food, for it is the fiber or "roughage" of bran that is so often missing from the typical Western diet and is so essential to proper digestion and elimination. Even the more traditional and conservative medical doctors are now recognizing the critical importance of fiber for the prevention of certain major diseases, and are recommending the addition of Miller's bran to the diet. Anyone who has been eating a typical high fat, low fiber diet and is eternally constipated as a result will benefit greatly by the simple addition of two tablespoons of bran to each meal. However, to avoid trouble with his digestive system, he should gradually increase the use of bran, starting with only two teaspoons a day. This may be sprinkled over foods, added to cereals or drinks, or baked into breads, casseroles, loaves, and so forth. Unfortunately, life is never simple—adding a little bran to your diet is only a partial solution at best. Prevention of bowel cancer, appendicitis, diverticulosis, varicose veins, and other such lovely benefits of the low fiber diet involves a more total dietary shift away from animal fats and processed foods to fruits, vegetables, and whole grains. But, for those who would rather do anything than give up their steak and Cool Whip, a little bran will certainly help to keep their bowels moving better. However, it should be mentioned that *too much fiber* can have drawbacks too. Although you will always get a natural balance of fiber from eating whole foods, the addition of too much bran, for example, may bind up certain critical nutrients like copper, iron, and zinc during digestion and prevent them from being assimilated.[1]

It is interesting that taking bran to lower blood cholesterol has been shown to be useless, whereas eating whole wheat, if it is hard wheat, will lower cholesterol 10 to 17 percent.[2]

Including bran in a diet is justified only in the case of elderly patients who are unable to chew their food and eat so little they are continuously constipated. Here bran is very helpful and the benefits clearly outweigh any drawbacks.

Bulgur

Bulgur is whole wheat that has been cracked into bits and parboiled, i.e., partially cooked. It requires very little cooking, in fact you can just soak it overnight and eat it cold, as in an increasingly popular Middle Eastern salad called *tabouleh*. Bulgur is almost as nutritious as whole wheat, but of course some nutrients are lost in cracking and cooking. Rancidity can be a problem, so give bulgur a good sniff before eating it.

Cracked Wheat

Cleverly named, cracked wheat is none other than whole wheat berries cracked into bits. Some nutrition is lost due to exposure of the inner layers, but it remains basically a sound food. It cooks up in about one-fourth the time of whole wheat and is often used in breads for added crunchiness.

Grits

Grits are tiny pieces of whole grains, somewhat smaller than cracked wheat. The most common are oat, corn, barley, and soy grits. All grits have the advantage of relatively short cooking times and work well in bread recipes. *Hominy grits* are still quite popular in the southern U.S., but they are not a whole food, since the hull and, usually, the germ of the corn have been removed.

Millet

Hulled millet cooks up in about 15 or 20 minutes and so is included here as a cereal, although it is as close to a whole grain as you can get, only the outer hull having been removed. As mentioned before, millet is by far one of the most nutritious grains, and makes an excellent breakfast mush.

Muesli

Muesli is Europe's version of granola. Made with grains, nuts, and dried fruit, it may be eaten cold with milk or cooked up like oatmeal.

Mush

"Mush" is just a new name for a lot of cereals mixed together, what used to be called porridge. Mushes may consist solely of various types of flakes, or have things like bran, soy grits, millet, buckwheat, and so forth added to them. Some makers of more elaborate mushes add raisins, dates, sunflower seeds, sesame seeds, walnuts, cashews, and just about anything else. Mushes cook up in 15 to 20 minutes and make a hearty breakfast dish that will keep you satisfied for many hours.

Oatmeal (Oat Flakes, Rolled Oats)

Long before kids' cereal bowls were filled with disguised sugar and red dye #40, oatmeal was the staple American breakfast, and still is in many rural areas of the country. As mentioned before, oatmeal is nothing more than whole oat groats that have been softened by steaming, flattened out, and dried. Some nutritional loss occurs but it remains a wholesome food. However, the paper-thin, "quick cooking" rolled oats should be avoided. Here the oat groat is cut up into smaller pieces and flattened out very thin so as to reduce cooking time. Much more nutritional loss is incurred and freshness may be doubtful.

Porridge

Simply a hot dish of one or more types of flakes, or coarsely ground grains (like cornmeal), porridge is often referred to as "mush" today. Adding nuts, seeds, or dried fruit, along with sweeteners and spices can make the variety of porridges endless.

Rice Polish

The outside layer of brown rice contains most of the grain's important nutrients, and polish is simply that layer ground into a flour-like consistency. Add it to mush mixtures and cereal dishes of all kinds to boost nutrition. Be aware, however, that it can go rancid rather easily and so is best purchased fresh and stored in the refrigerator.

Steel Cut Oats

Like cracked wheat, steel cut oats are the whole grain cracked into "grits." They cook up quickly, like oatmeal, but will have a firmer texture than the mush created by flakes.

Wheat Germ

Wheat germ is a natural food, but it is not a whole food. The "germ" of the wheat berry is the innermost core and one of the components which is sifted out when whole wheat becomes white flour. It contains a number of important nutrients, including the famous vitamin E, for which much money has been spent but little use has been found. Wheat germ is also a concentrated source of protein.

The most significant aspect of wheat germ, however, is some health devotees' obsession with it. Although there is nothing nutritional in wheat germ that you cannot easily obtain from other foods, many people feel it is something they simply cannot exist without. They put it in their granola, their pancakes, their breads, their salads, even their orange juice. Food manufacturers, particularly those producing packaged items for health food stores, have craftily cashed in on this obsession by boastingly adding wheat germ to everything from cereals to candy bars; every other shampoo, skin cream, and beauty soap has to have some form of wheat germ in it, as if this were a magic food, a fountain of youth.

All this would seem harmless if wheat germ had no intrinsic problems, but unfortunately it has a big one—rancidity. Because the major component of wheat germ is oil, and because unsaturated oils tend to oxidize and form peroxides when exposed to air, taking the germ out of the protective shell of the whole wheat kernel leaves it a prime target for rancidity, and rancidity is no small matter. The ingestion of rancid foods, which is remarkably common, is under suspicion as a cause of certain cancers, especially that of the stomach.

If, in spite of all this, you insist on eating wheat germ, try to obtain it as fresh as possible. Some stores make arrangements with local mills to have wheat germ delivered each week on the same day it is made. You may then purchase it fresh on that day and keep it refrigerated for a few days, after which, for longer storage it should be frozen. Other than this, nitrogen-flushed wheat germ—in which nitrogen gas (a natural component of air) has displaced the oxygen in the container—may be a safe alternative. It depends heavily upon how fresh the wheat germ was when it was packed, and how thorough the nitrogen flushing process was. I would be highly suspicious of "vacuum-packed" products. It is not usually a completely successful process. Never, never buy wheat germ that is loose or in ordinary packages unless it is at least refrigerated. It is claimed that *toasted wheat germ* will retain its freshness considerably longer than the raw, but of course that toasting process deteriorates some of the very nutritional properties you were eating wheat germ for in the first place.

I realize that I will not be pleasing a lot of friends in the health food industry with this little discourse, but wheat germ is a fragile food that perhaps was never meant to be isolated from the whole grain, and tendency toward rancidity is a bummer and just not worth the chance.

Incidentally, a new product, corn germ, is now appearing on the market in nitrogen flushed packages. Corn germ is a nice source of polyunsaturates and vitamin E, but certainly carries with it the same problems inherent in wheat germ.

Sugar, Sugar, and More Sugar

Nowhere is the deception practiced by advertisers touting the products which fill supermarket shelves more damaging than in the area of popular breakfast cereals. Manufacturers tear apart the whole grain, which has all the nutrition one could ever need, and discard its most nutritious parts; they artificially color and flavor, dose with chemical preservatives, and finally bombard with refined sugar what is left. After all this, a few synthetic vitamins are sprayed on, and suddenly this meager excuse for human food is magically transformed into a virtual power pack of energy and nutrition—one bowl each morning and you're on your way to eternal glowing health. Probably the only person who benefits from all this is your dentist. Here are just a few of the popular breakfast cereals and their sugar contents, expressed in terms of percentage of calories made up by sugar as compared to the total number of calories.

Sugar Content of Popular Cereals

Product	% Sucrose (White Sugar)
Cheerios	2.2
Post Toasties	4.1
Special K	4.4
Corn Flakes (Kellogg)	7.8
Raisin Bran (Kellogg)	10.6
Sugar Frosted Flakes	29.0
Frosted Mini Wheats	33.6
Sugar Pops	37.8
Cocoa Puffs	43.0
Cocoa Krispies	45.9
Trix	46.6
Froot Loops	47.4
Sugar Smacks	61.3

Source: Ira L. Shannon, Sucrose and Glucose Concentrations of Often Ingested Foods and Drinks. Dept. of Biochemistry, University of Texas Dental Branch, Houston, Texas.

As you can see you're often getting a lot more for your money than you expected. A healthy diet should have no more than 4 percent of its total calories from refined sugar. The average teenager may get up to 40 percent from refined sugar. Now, many entire books have been written about the negative effects sugar has upon health and there's no need to delve into them here. Suffice to say that it is a substance which all of us concerned with good nutrition should seek to minimize in our daily diets. Obviously, starting the day with a big bowl of Sugar Crunchies is not the right approach.

In addition to excessive sugar, commercial cereals usually contain one or more chemicals in the form of preservatives, artificial colors, or artificial flavors, and often are processed to the degree that much of the natural fiber is gone. Again, these are not necessary or desirable in the healthy diet.

But what about people who can't handle the blandness of oatmeal, porridge, or flakes for breakfast, no matter how disguised with raisins, honey, and spices? And what about those who simply have no time in the morning to mess around with cooking? For these people, the Creator has given us granola.

Granola

During the Civil War a ready-to-eat breakfast cereal consisting of little more than baked whole grain dough and called "Granula" was introduced. J. H. Kellogg, of Battle Creek fame, put together a cereal of baked oatmeal and whole grain dough he called "Granola," primarily as a good staple food for people committed to vegetarianism. The original granola waxed and waned in popularity but has recently been resurrected full force. Granola is now one of the most widely accepted "health foods," even among people who couldn't care less about what they eat, because, above all else, granola simply tastes good.

There are dozens of granola recipes and you surely will devise your own favorite after some experimenting, but the centerpoint of all granola is the mighty rolled oat. To this, most commercial granola makers add soy oil, wheat germ, honey, molasses, coconut, vanilla extract, sesame seeds, raisins, sunflower seeds. . . . The more exotic granolas contain blueberries, raspberries, orange oil, papaya, pineapple, dates, you name it. Here is a basic granola recipe you can begin with, and which we can modify somewhat to reduce some of the fats and sugars.

Basic Granola

6 cups rolled oats
1 cup unhulled sesame seeds
1 cup raw wheat germ
½ cup soy flour

1 cup soy oil (too much fat)
½ cup honey (too much sugar)
1 tsp. vanilla

Combine wet ingredients and dry ingredients separately and then mix together thoroughly. Spread out in a large roasting pan and bake at 225°F for 50–60 minutes, stirring occasionally.

As you can see, the two main problems here are fat and sugar. To make your granola stick together is going to require some oil, but a full cup in a recipe this size is unnecessary. I suggest mixing everything else together, then, start with a couple of tablespoons of oil or even liquid lecithin, a thick oil extracted from soybeans, blend until you get a consistency you can live with. All you're really concerned with is very lightly coating the grains so that they bake properly and adhere to each other somewhat.

The honey could also be reduced considerably, or better yet, eliminated entirely and replaced by chopped dates or raisins. If you prefer something syrupy like honey, try throwing dates or raisins in your blender with a little water and making a fruit puree which can then be used like honey or molasses. This kind of sweetener will contain all the natural fruit sugars plus the nutrients and fiber lacking in refined products like honey, molasses, or maple syrup.

After you've developed a basic granola you're satisfied with, try adding a few of the following optional ingredients to your recipe:

Nuts and Seeds	Fruits	Flavorings
raw sunflower seeds	raisins	cinnamon
raw pumpkin seeds	date pieces	nutmeg
flax seeds	dried apples	maple extract
sliced almonds	dehydrated blueberries	
raw cashew pieces	strawberries, raspberries	
diced walnuts		
raw peanuts		

How nutritious is granola anyway? Here's where I make more enemies. Any question as loaded as that one I always answer with another question: "Compared to what?" Compared to the sugar-coated plastic most children and many adults eat for breakfast, granola is great, and getting your family from processed cereals to granola will be a major step toward better health, particularly if you make your own and are in control of the ingredients. Store-bought varieties of granola contain a lot of oil and are 14 to 21 percent sugar. The important point, however, is that granola is basically a natural food that contains lots of natural fiber and no synthetic additives.

Comparing granola to say, whole grains, is another story. As we've already learned, rolled oats may suffer nutritional losses, wheat germ may be rancid (so may sunflower seeds for that matter), and granola contains lots of fat, both saturated (coconut) and unsaturated (soy oil). If you're on a low fat or low calorie diet, granola should be used carefully, or formulated accordingly. The combination of honey, molasses, coconut, and soy oil, along with nuts, seeds, and dried fruit, make granola a dieter's nightmare. After all, when you look over the ingredients, granola is nothing more than a crumbled up cookie without baking powder.

Granola may be eaten in the traditional fashion, in a bowl with milk, or simply as a dry snack. Either way granola is a perfect "transition" food to get the family away from the bad and toward the good. It is flavorful enough, sweet enough, and varied enough to be accepted by most people, no matter what their diet, and it at least helps to break the stereotype that all healthy foods are boring.

Selection and Storage

Since cereals are partially "processed," in that they have been fragmented or changed from the original whole grain, they are more vulnerable to spoilage than their parent grains, and so more attention should be paid to selection and storage.

Flakes and grits have a fairly good shelf life, and if you buy from a dealer who sells a lot of these, you probably will get a fresh product. Certainly the wariness with which you purchase wheat germ need not be exercised in buying these cereals. It wouldn't hurt though to give them a good sniff to see if they smell stale or even "musty" (a sign of developing mold). Flakes are also especially popular with moths, so you might keep an eye out for developing larvae. This is no reflection on the freshness of the flakes, just unpleasant for most of us.

As mentioned already, granola has a somewhat higher rancidity potential than plain cereal grains due to the presence of wheat germ, oil and certain seeds. Usually a sniff or two will cue you to freshness, but the ultimate test is taste: a distinct burning in the back of the throat a few moments after eating.

Flakes, grits, and granolas that will not be consumed in a couple of weeks time should be kept refrigerated. Wheat germ, corn germ, and rice polish should be frozen unless they can be consumed in a few days, but always at least refrigerated. "Whole" cereals like millet and buckwheat may be stored without refrigeration for months.

Preparation

The general rule for all flakes, grits, mushes, and hulled grains like buckwheat and millet is two parts water to one part cereal, bring to a boil, turn to low, cover, and cook 15 to 20 minutes or until water is absorbed and cereal is tender. If you're concerned about energy conservation or simply want to save time in the morning, combine water and cereal at night and let soak until morning—they'll cook up in just a few minutes this way.

Lots of goodies can be added to plain oatmeal or other flakes and grit mixtures. Try dried fruits like raisins, chopped dates, chopped figs, and soaked prunes, or spice it up with cinnamon, allspice, nutmeg, cloves, or vanilla. Adding a few sunflower or pumpkin seeds will give some crunchiness to the mushy texture. And don't overlook the obvious—fresh fruit. Berries and slices of fresh apples, pears, peaches, papaya, and bananas all turn the lowly mush into a treat.

Incidentally, flakes and mush mixes are great foods for camping, since they conserve fuel and require no special storage. Their light weight makes them excellent for backpacking, and they provide the most needed nutrient for that type of strenuous activity: carbohydrate.

Recipes

Tabouli (one of many spellings)[3]

1½ cups bulgur
3 cups vegetable stock or water
1 tsp. salt
½ cup cooked white beans
2 tomatoes, chopped
3 Tbps. olive oil
pepper to taste

pinch garlic
2 Tbsp. chopped chives
2 tsp. chopped mint
juice of 2 lemons
¼ cup chopped parsley
lettuce

Bring salted stock to a boil. Add bulgur, bring to a second boil, remove from heat, cover, and set aside for 1 hour. Drain excess water and chill the grain. Toss with all remaining ingredients, taste for seasoning, and serve on lettuce bed. Serves 6.

All-Grain Mush

3 cups rolled oats
1 cup soy flakes (or grits)
1 cup rye flakes
1 cup wheat flakes
½ cup bran
½ cup bulgur
½ cup raw buckwheat groats

Mix all ingredients together and store in refrigerator. As a breakfast cereal, use one part mixture to two parts water. Bring to a boil, turn heat low and simmer 15–20 minutes or until all water is absorbed. Add fruit or sweetener.

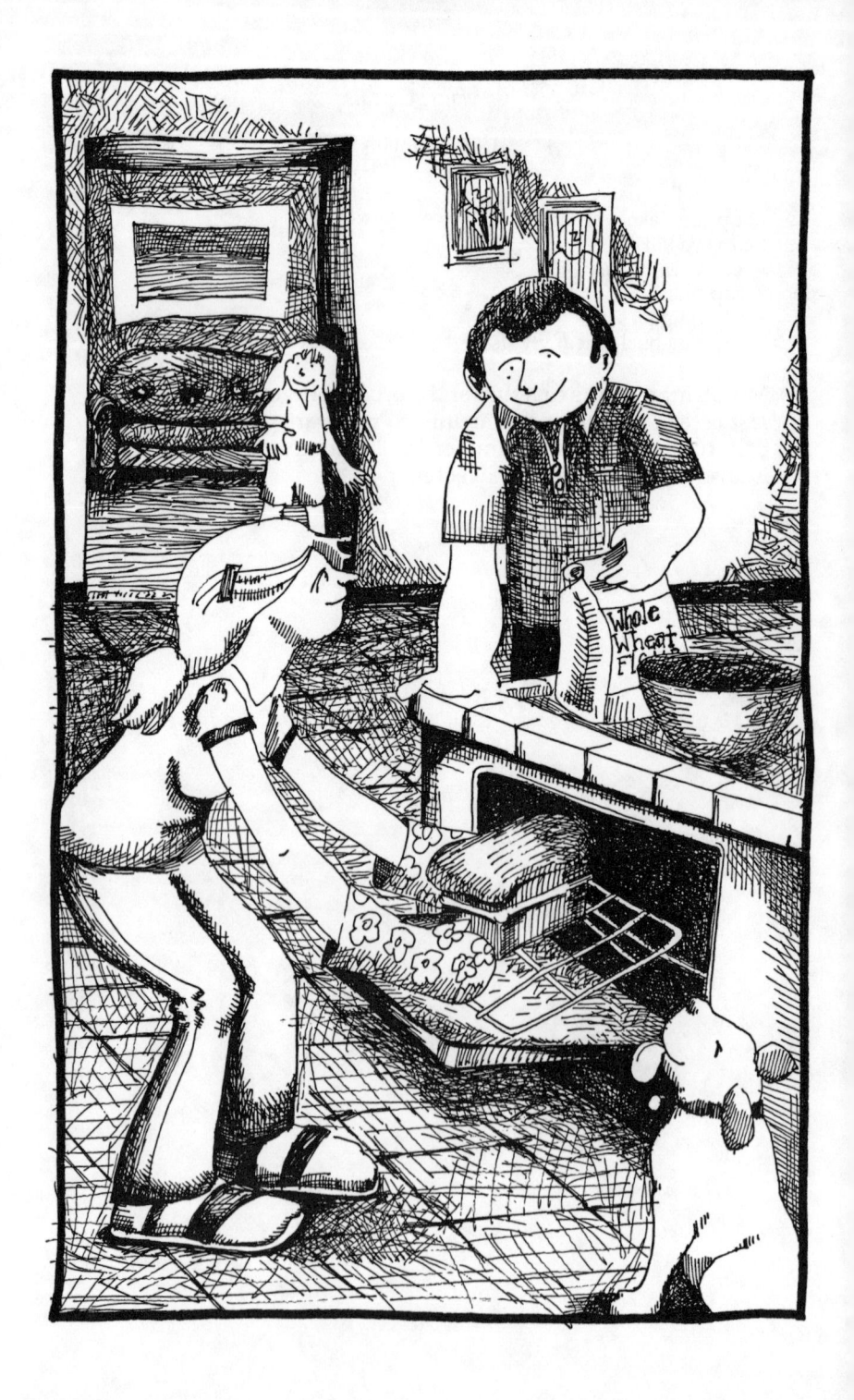

CHAPTER 9

Flour, Baked Goods, and Pasta

Although I highly recommend eating grains in their whole, natural state, I'm realistic enough to know that most people are not about to sit down to a big bowl of wheat berries too often. All but the most stoical among us will no doubt continue to take our grains in the form of bread, pasta, and baked goods in general. And this is not bad news by any means. A loaf of home-baked bread made from freshly milled grains and other natural ingredients or a steaming plate of whole wheat spaghetti is an excellent staple in any good diet. Although texture and taste may vary, a good home cook can produce any bread, cake, cookie, or pastry out of whole grain flour and natural sweeteners that could be made with white flour and white sugar. These products will retain much of the vitamins, minerals, and proteins of the whole grain and all the fiber.

For those with neither the time nor the inclination for home baking, the natural food industry markets a huge variety of ready-to-eat breads and bakery products. We shall examine many of these for quality and general desirability in the diet.

Flour

If I had to pick a single food to symbolize all that is wrong with modern man's perversion of nature, it would be white flour. Not because white flour is all that destructive to the human system, certainly tobacco and alcohol rank much higher in that contest; but because the motivations behind the production, marketing, and widespread public acceptance of white flour are so patently representative of the type of unenlightened thinking that has led us so far down the path toward ecological chaos.

Man's infatuation with refined flour emerged along with his infatuation with all things refined, aristocratic, and non-peasant. When the rich and royal of centuries past sought to separate themselves from the common man they did so in all facets of their lives: in the houses they lived in, the clothes they wore, their speech, their mannerisms, and in the food they ate. While the lowly serf was happy to have enough coarse wheat or corn to make bread for his family, the idle rich man indulged himself in wasteful amounts of meats, sweets, and butterfat. Somewhere around this time, the first loaf of white bread appeared on some nobleman's table, and its airy, soft texture was a welcome diversion from the jaw-breaking bricks from peasant ovens. A new fetish was born.

Man seems to have a natural desire to emulate the affluent, and it is a mixed blessing indeed. Although this striving for upward mobility may be the very seed of progress, it rests on the false assumption that because a person is rich he somehow knows what's good. At any length, as the 20th century approached, white bread became the symbol of all that was rich, modern, and refined. Whole wheat bread was for common laborers and dumb farmers.

The loaf of white bread you see in most households today is the end product of a long series of "advances" in bread making. Today's children put their peanut butter and jelly on a spongy combination of chemical dough stiffeners and conditioners, mold-retarding preservatives, yeast nutrients, sugar, hydrogenated oil, refined bleached white flour, and air—lots of air. Take a loaf of supermarket white bread and crush it together in your hands until it's as solid as you can get it. With all the air displaced you don't have much left in your hands do you? Such is the price of progress, and profit margins.

The main commercial rationales for white flour in today's marketplace are that it doesn't spoil easily and it doesn't get infested with insects. That's pretty easy to believe. There's really very little left in it to spoil by the time refinement is complete, and it has so little taste and nutrition that its not worth any self-respecting weevil's efforts. Virtually everything worth eating has been discarded in the refinement process, leaving carbohydrate, some protein, and only minimal amounts of vitamins and minerals. Look at the difference between whole wheat and ordinary all-purpose white flour:

Nutrient Values of Whole Wheat and White Flour

per 100 grams (3½ ounces)	Calories	Protein (grams)	Total Carbohydrate (grams)	Fiber (grams)	Calcium (milligrams)	Phosphorus (milligrams)	Iron (milligrams)	Potassium (milligrams)	Vitamin B_1 (milligrams)	Vitamin B_2 (milligrams)	Niacin (milligrams)
Whole Wheat	330	14	69.1	2.3	36	383	3.1	370	.57	.12	4.3
White Flour	364	10.5	76.1	0.3	16	87	0.8	95	.08	.06	1.0

Source: U.S. Dept. of Agriculture Handbook no. 8.

As you can easily see, there is considerable loss of nutrition, and this is by no means the complete story. About twenty nutrients are removed during processing, many of them important trace elements not routinely tested for in typical food analyses, but nevertheless critical to the balance of nutrients in natural food *and* in the human system. And here I feel lies the most important issue of all—this question of balance. Is the human body a simple "warehouse" for nutrients, which must be kept "in stock" to be used for its ongoing activities? Do we merely have a minimum daily requirement for forty or so elements which must be acquired from our food at random and put into inventory? And does it really matter where these elements come from as long as we get them?

The idea that an organism as incredibly sophisticated as the human body would operate by taking in food of any kind, breaking it down, absorbing only those nutrients it needed and discarding the rest seems absurdly simplistic to me. The balance of nutrients, the relationship they have to each other, must play a role in the way the body reacts to food. Perhaps one nutrient is only absorbed in the presence of another and in some critical proportion to it. The carburetor in your automobile runs on a mixture of air and gasoline. Giving it air at 9 a.m. and gasoline at noon won't get you out of the garage: they have to be given simultaneously and in proper proportion to each other. Now, your car may *run* if the proportions are off by some measure, but it won't run well or efficiently. Perhaps the same sort of situation exists in your body, but of course on a far more complicated level. Eating enough refined food and popping a few vitamin pills may provide your body with all the nutrients it needs to "get by," but to work efficiently and at its optimum it may need those nutrients in better proportion to each other and may also require trace amounts of micronutrients unavailable in refined foods.

"Getting by" seems to be the state of most peoples' bodies. "Getting by" means a couple of colds a year, an occasional infection of some kind, an allergy or two perhaps, pasty skin, brittle hair, indigestion, headaches, constipation, running out of energy midway through the day, irritability, dependency on sweets, and you can fill in the rest. Sound like people you know? All these ordinary, accepted maladies are simply signs of bigger things to come. It's your body trying to tell you to shape up or it will ship you out. These people come running to doctors and even health food stores when they're in their fifties or younger and are suddenly facing diabetes, arthritis, a heart attack or cancer. When your car has a heart attack you can always get a new one.

My point is simple: eat your foods the way Nature made them, and the nutrients will be in the correct proportions to each other. The closer you stay to this ideal, the better your health will be. The farther you get from it, the more trouble you're asking for.

The Fallacy of Enrichment

No phrase more deserves enclosure in quotation marks than "enriched white flour," for the enrichment is only a figure of speech. When white flour's nutritional deficiencies were revealed, government agencies, fearing outbreaks of deficiency-related diseases like beri-beri and pellagra if the population derived too great a percentage of their calories from this half-food, initiated the policy of enrichment. Flour producers were instructed to offer a version of white flour with nutrients added back into it. Synthetic nutrients, produced in a laboratory, were sprayed onto the flour like paint. Now, for all we know synthetic nutrients may be as good as the real thing, and enrichment may be a valid way of restoring vitamins and minerals lost during processing, except that the enrichers didn't even come close to putting back what they took out. About twenty nutrients are removed but only four or five may be added back, usually iron, thiamine (vitamin B1), riboflavin (vitamin B2), and niacin. Sodium may be added but only because salt is used in the recipe for flavor. This is enrichment? Pardon me as I squeeze one more drop from a well-worn analogy, but this kind of enrichment is like the thief who steals everything you own, then gives you back $10 and calls you "enriched." Thanks a lot.

Nutrient Values of Whole Wheat and Enriched White Flour

per 100 grams (3½ ounces)	Calories	Protein (grams)	Total Carbohydrate (grams)	Fiber (grams)	Calcium (milligrams)	Phosphorus (milligrams)	Iron (milligrams)	Potassium (milligrams)	Vitamin B₁ (milligrams)	Vitamin B₂ (milligrams)	Niacin (milligrams)
Whole Wheat	330	14.0	69.1	2.3	36	383	3.1	370	.57	.12	4.3
Enriched White Flour	364	10.5	76.1	0.3	16	87	2.9	95	.44	.26	3.5

Source: U.S. Dept. of Agriculture Handbook no. 8.

As you can see, even among the relatively few nutrients measured in this U.S. Dept. of Agriculture analysis, "enriched white flour" comes out a hands down loser.

As we have seen before, the most important substance missing from a refined food is often simple fiber. Attempts are lately being made by large commercial bread producers to add fiber back into their products, and they are advertising that fact heavily. But their concept of "natural fiber" is most curious: one company uses wood fiber in their bread. True, it's natural, but to what, termites? Are we very far from the day when synthetic fiber will begin appearing in bread?

Whole Wheat Flour

Despite this good sense and logic, white bread will continue to be a major part of the American diet for a long time to come, but it need not be part of yours. Whole grain breads are widely available, even in many supermarkets, and are simple to make at home. The first step obviously is whole wheat flour.

You can get whole wheat flour in a number of ways: buy it prepackaged in a supermarket or health food store, buy it in bulk or freshly ground at a natural food store or co-op, or grind it yourself. As with all things in life, there are good and bad points to each choice.

The convenience of grabbing a nice neat package of flour off the shelf in your local market as you're zipping up the aisle looking for squeezable toilet paper is a temptation, but not recommended. Unless you live in an extremely enlightened area where whole wheat flour is purchased as often as bananas, that crisp little bag of flour is probably as old as the store. Also, you should know that whole wheat flour is not necessarily free of additives. Chemicals like potassium bromate are often added as conditioning agents.

Flour at your nearby health food store may not be much fresher, especially if it is primarily a vitamin shop. Remember that the whole wheat berry contains an unsaturated oil that can easily go rancid, and grinding it into flour obviously exposes that oil to its arch enemy, oxygen. Any untreated flour sitting on a shelf at room temperature for more than a few days is suspect. It won't kill you, but rancidity has begun and if you want fresh food, this isn't the best way to go about it.

Natural food stores selling flour in bulk may purchase it from a local mill, buy name brand flour like Arrowhead Mills or El Molino from their regional distributor, or grind it themselves. The best way to find out about freshness and quality is to ask. Is it from a local mill? How often does it come in? How often do they grind their wheat and how often do you get it? What day does it come it? How do you store it? These are all valid questions, and although they may put you on the proprietor's Top Ten Pests list, he should respect your right to have this information. If the store grinds its own grain on the premises, you can easily find out when the grinding is done and make it your business to get flour fresh that day. Larger stores are simply too busy to grind flour to order; but they generally grind flour once a day to keep their bulk bins full, so you're still getting a fairly fresh product.

Smaller natural food stores often own mills that can produce up to 25 pounds an hour and will grind many flours fresh to the customer's order. This is obviously the best way to get whole grain flour. If you take it home and use it that day, or store it in your refrigerator for up to a week or so, you can be sure you've gotten the freshest product available. If it is inconvenient for you to run to the store each week for flour, you can always buy a month's supply or more and freeze it. Freezing will not harm the flavor significantly and will prevent rancidity totally, although it will destroy vitamin E. It will also, incidentally, kill any little insects that may be in there growing. Finally, for the true fanatic, owning your own mill is the ultimate guarantee of freshness. You can grind your flour just before baking and make only what you need. Manually operated models range from $20 to $120 and electric ones from $250 to $500. Mills are discussed in more detail in Chapter 20.

Stone Grinding

"Stone ground whole wheat flour" is one of those catchy phrases you hear and see so often in the natural food business. It refers simply to the milling of grain by grinding it between two "stones," one stationary and one movable. These stones are not the type you would cast through a window, but a special type of stone selected and designed specifically for milling. The two flat-surfaced stones are set close together, and as grain passes between them it is broken down to any texture from a cracked cereal to a fine pastry flour depending upon how closely the stones are spaced.

The advantage of stone grinding is the lower temperatures at which the flour is kept. A good stone grinder should not bring grain temperature above 90° F or so, since higher temperatures result in the breakdown and destruction of nutrients, especially vitamin E and the enzymes natural to the grain. The alternative method of milling, with steel plates or rollers, brings temperatures way above this level and much is lost in the process. This is the chosen technique of the large commercial grain processors since stone grinding is much more troublesome than steel.

A reasonable question at this point is whether the advantage of lower milling temperatures, is not lost when you cook the flour, at temperatures of 350° F or more. After all, nobody eats raw flour, so why worry about delicate enzymes and vitamins that are going to be destroyed in the oven anyhow? If you're buying your flour freshly milled and using it right away, or if you mill your own at home and use it immediately, it probably doesn't make any real difference. It's in the preservation or shelf life of the flour that these nutrients play their major role. Vitamin E is any oil's first line of defense against rancidity, and if a whole wheat flour still has its vitamin E intact because it was milled at a low temperature, it has a far better chance of staying fresh on the shelf for a while. Also, although this business of enzymes has yet to be fully investigated, I strongly suspect that the natural enzymes in any plant food serve as a superior defense against spoilage. Experience in the natural food business has shown me time and time again that many cooked foods (e.g., roasted nuts) spoil much faster than raw ones, particularly if they contain a lot of unsaturated oil.

Other Flours

Almost everyone's first excursion into natural food baking is via whole wheat flour, but there are lots of other whole grain flours available, many freshly ground, which can be easily used to add great variety to your baking repertoire. Any whole grain, and many beans, may be made into flour.

One that you should become aware of quickly is *whole wheat pastry flour*. Pastry flour is ground from the soft variety of wheat and is particularly suitable when baking without yeast, i.e., with baking powder or soda, but does not work all that well with yeast. Pie crusts, cakes, cookies, and pancakes are among the foods suited to pastry flour.

Rye flour of course is great for breads, imparting its own distinctive flavor. (If caraway seeds are added for additional taste, it is called pumpernickel.) Occasionally a recipe calls for *dark rye flour*. This is just another way of saying whole rye flour, flour that has not been bolted (i.e., sifted) to remove any of the bran or germ. As with most flours other than wheat, rye does not have a great deal of rising power by itself and usually has to be mixed with some type of wheat flour to produce the lighter textures most people want. I have tasted German rye bread made exclusively with rye and a sourdough culture. It feels like a block of lead but if sliced paper thin is truly delicious.

Cornmeal should be a working part of any whole grain baker's kitchen stock. The rich taste and texture of cornbread and corn muffins are enough to win over even the most devoted junk food addict. Some people distinguish between *cornmeal*, a coarser, grittier grind better suited for tortillas and the like, and *corn flour*, finer textured and better for breads. Names aside, it is best to decide the texture you want and get corn ground accordingly, if possible.

The cornmeal found in supermarkets is usually "degerminated." The corn germ has been removed to prevent spoilage to some degree. Unfortunately, a good deal of the nutritional value has also been removed. "Bolted" cornmeal has been sifted to remove most of the bran (fiber), yet the germ is left intact. Neither of these is desirable if whole cornmeal is available.

Soy flour is basically ground up soybeans. It is useful because of its high protein value and the fact that so many people are allergic to wheat. Soy flour is found in a number of forms: defatted, toasted and raw. The defatted and full-fat forms can be used interchangeably in any recipe, and the decision pretty much depends on your own feeling about oil in the diet. If you're shooting for a low fat, low oil (same thing) diet, then a defatted flour would be your choice. Raw soy flour is fine for long baking but should not be used uncooked or in foods only cooked slightly, since the soybean contains certain toxic elements which interfere with protein digestion, among other things.

Unbleached white flour will usually be available in natural food stores primarily because it is called for so often in recipes. It is by no means a whole food and really no different than ordinary all-purpose white flour except that it has not gone through the final bleaching stage of refinement. Its nutritional value is low and if it has any advantage over bleached white flour it is in the absence of the chemicals used for bleaching. However, it is a useful "transition" aid for people switching over to whole grain baking. Many people accustomed to the airy, spongy texture of white bread initially find whole grain breads too coarse for their liking. Mixing whole wheat flour with unbleached white flour provides a sort of compromise. The resulting bread is heavier and grainier than white bread but not to the point that it is totally rejected by the new initiate. So, for the mother trying to ease her husband and children into whole foods, this compromise bread is a good vehicle, much like the brown rice mixed in with the white or the bran sneaked into the standard breakfast cereal. At least some genuine nutrition is present in the whole wheat part of the compromise, and a good deal of fiber is added to the diet. Gradually the proportion of white flour can be lessened, and before long the gang will be wolfing down that old health food bread like troopers.

Gluten flour is often used by bakers who want to get extra rising power in their bread. Gluten is a protein in wheat, and also the part that traps the gases produced by yeast and thus allows bread to rise. You generally won't find 100 percent gluten flour available, but a mixture of gluten and white flour which is easier to work with. Gluten flour is especially useful when you are baking with specialty flours like buckwheat, millet, or rice, which by themselves don't have great rising potential. The massaging of dough known as *kneading* is what develops and conditions the gluten so that it will do its thing when the baking begins.

Carob flour, more commonly called *carob powder*, is becoming increasingly popular as a substitute for cocoa and chocolate. It is far lower in fat and calories than chocolate, and does not contain any of the harmful compounds like methylxanthine or caffeine common to chocolate. In addition it contains more natural sugars, fiber, and minerals than either cocoa or chocolate.

Carob powder is ground from the pods of the carob tree, which grows in many areas of the world, the best, however, being grown in the area around the Mediterranean. Carob, also known as St. John's Bread, is eaten whole by people in this area and is said to resemble the taste of fresh dates.

When substituting carob powder for cocoa, use an equal amount called for in the recipe. When substituting for chocolate, use three tablespoons of carob powder plus one tablespoon of water for each square of chocolate. Since carob powder is 46 percent natural sugar, less sweetener should be used than when using cocoa or unsweetened chocolate.

Both raw and roasted forms of carob powder may be available in natural food stores. The raw is preferable for baking since you're going to cook it anyway and there's no point in cooking it twice. It will be more flavorful when cooked for the first time. Roasted carob powder is generally used for mixing in liquids to produce carob flavored drinks, hot or cold. It is a good substitute for hot cocoa or for chocolate flavoring in milk shakes and smoothies.

Although carob is primarily used in sweets like brownies, cookies, and cakes, I have seen breads made with carob flour conbined with other flours as well.

Lots of other flours are usually available for natural food baking, although some may be hard to find in certain areas. Besides the major flours we've discussed so far you will eventually find recipes calling for barley flour, triticale flour, rice flour, millet flour, oat flour, buckwheat flour, pea flour, and garbanzo bean flour. Each of these has its own special values and limitations, and it's interesting to experiment with all of them.

If you're fortunate enough to live near a store that has a mill and will grind your flour to order, you can obtain most of these flours fresh. If it is a stone mill, which it probably will be, certain flours cannot be made. Oats, for example, have a high fat and moisture content and thus tend to clog stone mills readily unless the grain has been oven dried in advance. Corn is also a problem for small mills, since the kernels are so hard they tend to pit the stones quickly. Rather than replace an expensive set of grinding stones every couple of months, most mill owners decline to grind corn. The alternative is a steel mill specifically for corn, and if the store's demand for fresh cornmeal is sufficient, they may have one. Much the same holds true for garbanzo flour, the beans being too large and too hard for a stone mill to handle efficiently without damage.

Organic Flours

Stores will sometimes offer the consumer a choice between flours ground from organically grown grains or the commercial variety, at least in the case of whole wheat. More often than not, many of their other flours may only be available in the organic form, since that may be all the local distributor carries. And if the store is grinding its own flour, it is often easier to obtain organic rye, corn, triticale, etc., than to keep a consistent supply of commercially grown grains. Regardless, whether or not you want to buy organic flour for your baking is totally up to you and how you feel personally about pesticides and artificial fertilizers. Organic flour will not taste any better, or possess any superior nutritional benefits, other than the absence of chemical additives, although you should be aware that a product may legally be labelled "organically grown" and still contain pesticides.

Selection and Storage

Common sense tells us that the more a food is broken down into smaller pieces, the more surfaces are exposed to air and the faster spoilage will occur. Sliced carrots spoil faster than whole carrots, but grated carrots spoil even faster than sliced; chopped meat will spoil faster than a side of beef. It is this unrelenting law of the universe that makes flour the most vulnerable form of whole grains, and makes your selection and storage of it critical.

The degree and rate of spoilage for a given type of flour depend largely on its fat content. High oil flours like wheat, rye, rice, corn, and full-fat soy require greater care than unbleached white, gluten, and defatted soy. The importance of buying your flour as fresh as possible was discussed earlier. Once purchased flour should be refrigerated quickly. Refrigeration will slow down the rate of spoilage sufficiently to keep it relatively stable for a few weeks, but longer storage should be in the freezer.

As with whole grains, if you should find weevils in your flour and you choose to deal with them rather than waste flour, a 72-hour freeze will kill them, and a quick sifting will remove the deceased from your future bread.

Leavening

There are two types of leavening or "rising" agents commonly used in baking: those which depend upon the behavior of live micro-organisms, like yeast and sourdough cultures, and those which rely on a gas producing chemical reaction, like baking soda and powder.

Yeast

Baking yeast or active yeast, not to be confused with brewer's yeast or "nutritional yeast" (discussed in Chapter 18), is used primarily for breads, but occasionally for pancakes, muffins, and cakes, even pizza crusts. Active dry yeast should be purchased in small amounts and kept refrigerated once opened. There should be a date on the package and the yeast may not be very useful after that date. Natural food stores usually carry active yeast in small envelopes, generally three hooked together, or in 4-ounce, 8-ounce, or 16-ounce foil packages. Red Star and El Molino are two good brands to look for. Some supermarket brands contain preservatives, so be sure to check the label if that concerns you.

Yeast should always be dissolved in warm water (110°–115°F) before using. It is best to use a thermometer to verify the water temperature, since yeast is easily destroyed in hot liquids. Many a loaf of good bread has been ruined simply because the yeast was killed.

Remember that yeast may only be used with hard wheat flours, not with the softer pastry wheats. Hard wheat, with its high protein content, is the only grain with sufficient gluten to trap the gases produced by yeast and induce rising. Other grains like rye, barley, soy, and so forth have to be mixed with hard wheat flour or gluten flour if you expect them to rise well with yeast. Otherwise you must use baking powder or soda.

Sourdough

In the old days, a lump of dough from a batch prepared for bread was saved and allowed to ferment, giving rise to yeast-like organisms, which could then be used to "start" a new batch of dough. Sourdough cultures were often perpetuated indefinitely and even passed on in families, the result being that today many such cultures are over a century old, and highly treasured like vintage wines. Stores often sell little packets of sourdough culture you can use to start your own family treasure. Be aware that successful sourdough breads depend heavily on local climate conditions, the area around San Francisco often is heralded as the best in the U.S. It may not be as easy to produce top quality sourdough bread in Phoenix or Denver.

Baking soda

Baking soda is the common name for sodium bicarbonate or bicarbonate of soda, a chemical compound produced by combining soda ash and carbon dioxide. It is a leavening agent used in so-called quick breads, which do not require kneading and rising before baking, but mainly in cookies, cakes, pies, pancakes, and any other baked goods using pastry wheat flours or flours other than hard wheat.

Bicarbonate of soda is a strong alkali and as such is believed to destroy many of the B-complex vitamins in wheat flour. For this reason it is avoided by some.

Baking powder

There are a number of varieties of baking powder, but all contain baking soda as a major ingredient. Some contain cream of tartar while others have monocalcium phosphate, sodium phosphate, or sodium aluminum sulphate. All will yield an alkaline residue in the body and thus be harmful to B vitamins, but the least destructive of these is the combination of baking soda and monocalcium phosphate used in at least two major brands, Rumford and Fleischmann's. Those containing sodium aluminum sulphate are viewed with concern by some, since excessive amounts of aluminum in the body are not desirable; however, it appears that this substance is not absorbed after reacting in the system.

Some recipes call for "double acting" baking powder. These contain both monocalcium phosphate and sodium aluminum phosphate as well as baking soda, and are designed to rise more, due to the presence of two rising agents.

Flavors and Textures

A number of products for creating various flavors and textures in baked goods are sold in natural food stores. Some of the common ones deserve mention here.

Bran

Wheat bran is an excellent source of dietary fiber. Since it is mostly indigestible, it provides no other significant nutrition but lends the pleasantly coarse texture to bran muffins and coarse bran breads. Keep in mind, however, that bran tends to deplete the body's store of certain important minerals and so should be used judiciously.

Bran is cheap and rarely spoils. I have seen it in pretty boxes for up to $2 a pound in supermarkets and as low as 15 or 20 cents a pound in bulk food stores. Take your pick.

Coconut

Dried coconut, or dessicated coconut as it is formally titled, is called for in lots of baking recipes for both flavor and texture. It can be purchased in a variety of forms, granulated, shredded, and sliced, as well as in a number of sizes. It is expensive when you look at the per pound price, but it is so light that it actually adds little cost to your baking. People concerned with saturated fats in their diets should be aware that coconut is the highest in this category, even higher than meat, cheese, and eggs. Anyone on a low fat diet for medical reasons should scrupulously avoid coconut and its products.

Since coconut is high in fat, it will spoil, though not easily since the oil is saturated. You should store it in a relatively cool place, however, to keep it fresh for any length of time.

Kelp

Kelp is a seaweed found mainly in the Pacific Ocean, although some of the best kelp is supposed to come from the cold waters around Norway. Kelp is dried and ground into a powder and sold in natural food stores as a "salt substitute" of sorts. It does of course contain salt of its own since it grows all its life in salt water, but adds a strong flavor to foods while not adding a great deal of salt to the diet. Kelp is more often used in soups and salad dressings but is occasionally called for in baking recipes. It has no real spoilage problems.

Powdered Milk

Natural food stores sell non-instant powdered milk. This may be reconstituted into milk simply by adding water (four parts water to one part milk powder) or used dry in recipes. The term "non-instant" means that it will not dissolve freely into a glass of water just by stirring it around. Instant milk powders are processed for each mixing. Non-instant milk is simply fresh milk that has been spray-dried and so requires a little more effort to dissolve. Putting the milk and water into a blender at a low speed for a minute or so will do the trick, but a good vigorous shaking in a bottle will work just as well. Usually nonfat or skim, as well as whole milk, is sold. Nonfat is by far the most popular for use in baking recipes and for homemade yogurt (see Chapter 14).

Dry milk won't spoil readily unless it gets moisture in it. I have seen it sold loose in bulk bins successfully in drier climates, but in moister areas it should be packaged to keep humidity out. As long as you keep it dry you may buy in larger quantities safely.

Sea Salt

Let's get something straight right here: salt is salt whether it comes from the ground or the sea, and if you're on a sodium restricted diet or just realize the potential harm in adding salt to your diet, sea salt should be avoided as carefully as salt from the box with the little girl and her umbrella. Actually, all salt is sea salt, since it all came from the sea.

If you wish to use salt in cooking, certain differences between sea salt and ordinary commercial salt may interest you. Table salt is processed to some degree and certain nutrients are removed. Additives may be incorporated to prevent caking and keep the salt flowing freely. Sea salt is just dehydrated sea water and contains all of the natural sea minerals; about one-third of it is minerals other than sodium chloride.

Incidentally, don't be intimidated into using salt in baking just because a recipe calls for it. Salt performs no function in the recipe, but is simply for taste. Most people are so accustomed to and overstimulated by the taste of salt in their foods that anything without it tastes like pillow stuffing. Try doing without it for two weeks and see how sensitive your taste buds become. Salt is merely an unnecessary stimulant, and you may eliminate it from any recipe without affecting the basic quality of the finished product.

If you find your food tragically boring without salt, see Chapter 15 for a number of "salt substitutes" that will add flavors to your diet.

Vanilla

Vanilla extract is a derivative of the vanilla bean. It contains ethyl alcohol and often glycerin, propylene glycol, sugar, and corn syrup. Natural food stores often carry a product labelled "Pure Vanilla Extract." This should mean that it is only vanilla and alcohol and no other additives. Using the scrapings from inside whole vanilla bean pods is the only way to avoid the alcohol, which disappears during cooking anyhow.

You may, incidentally, make your own vanilla extract quite easily by soaking sliced vanilla beans in brandy or vodka for about two weeks; shake once a day.

Supermarkets sell *vanillin*, a synthetic flavoring often made from the waste products of the wood pulp industry. Large doses have been known to kill mice.

Occasionally you will stumble upon recipes calling for other extracts, like that of almond, walnut, or orange. These should be available in "pure" form, again meaning alcohol plus the derivative.

Packaged Baked Goods

The age of convenience is solidly upon us, and it would be naive of me to think that everyone is going to run out and buy flour and yeast and start baking his own bread. Many will, of course, and be pleasantly rewarded for their efforts, but for the majority, picking up a loaf of bread in the market will remain the prime source. And this is not nearly as bad an alternative as it used to be. As little as ten years ago it was hard to find a good loaf of bread made from whole wheat and other natural ingredients that hadn't been frozen for four years. The market for wholesome foods was small then, and no bakery could possibly survive baking fresh "health bread" more than once a month. But all that has changed, and demands have increased enough to make whole grain baking not only profitable but highly competitive in many areas.

Many large commercial bakers are getting into the natural bread business, or at least trying to, and healthful breads are beginning to appear in major supermarkets everywhere. I advise you, however, to be a little cautious about snapping one of these off the shelf and assuming the best ingredients are used. As we are all painfully aware, modern merchandising is not above using deception to sell a product. Many breads that appear to be full of whole grain goodness and Nature's foods are merely designed and packaged to look that way. Fortunately, we have labeling laws in this country that, although not strict enough to my way of thinking, demand a certain degree of truth in advertising and packaging. So, although the label may be misleading, somewhere in small print you will find an official list of ingredients. By regulation this list should give all ingredients in descending order of their proportions. In other words, the ingredient that is used most in the recipe must be listed first, and so on. If you pick up a loaf of bread that purports to be "100% natural" and full of "whole grain goodness" and of course with "no preservatives," you might easily be persuaded that you are buying a bread made from whole wheat flour and other wholesome products. In fact, a review of the label may reveal the prime ingredient to be unbleached enriched white flour with a little whole wheat thrown in somewhere along the line. You may also be surprised to find white sugar, brown sugar, corn syrup, and hydrogenated oils, none of which you really had in mind when you bought the bread. This is not to say that you won't find a real loaf of whole natural bread, with no undesirable ingredients, in a supermarket, nor can you be guaranteed that the bread you buy in a health food store is free from processed ingredients. All I'm saying is that in both cases you should take a minute to check over the label and be sure you're getting what you want.

A basic loaf of good bread could contain as few as three ingredients: whole wheat flour, water, and yeast. It is unlikely, however, that you will see bread this simple being sold in stores, for it is too bland for most peoples' tastes. Usually store bread contains at least whole wheat flour (which may or may not be stoneground), some kind of oil (usually soy or safflower), honey and/or molasses, yeast, and salt. This is still fairly basic, and the more popular breads these days are multigrain, often containing nine, ten, or even twelve different whole grains ground together. Other ingredients that may be thrown in are gluten flour (to increase rising), raisin syrup (a sweetener), and cracked wheat, bran, soy grits, or rolled oats, for texture. Most of these make for more flashiness than nutrition, however, and a simple whole wheat bread is as good as any.

Ingredients you want to avoid are any kind of white flour, be it enriched or unbleached; hydrogenated or partially hydrogenated oils of any kind, palm oil, coconut oil, cottonseed oil; sugar, brown sugar, raw sugar, turbinado sugar, yellow-d sugar, corn syrup, invert syrup, fructose, sucrose; and of course the more obvious additives like BHA, BHT, EDTA, sodium propionate, and various dough conditioners. None of this last group is likely to appear in a whole grain bread but it never hurts to check.

Also, watch out for any bread which lists its first ingredient as "wheat flour." Since white flour is processed from wheat, this may mean nothing more than good old white flour. The word "natural" has no legal definition, so it can be freely applied to white sugar or white flour. Advertising a product as 100 percent natural means little other than that it is free of synthetic additives.

Although whole wheat is customarily the base for breads, you will also run across breads made from practically every conceivable combination of grains. Some of these are designed specifically for people with particular food allergies—soy-millet bread, for example, is purchased largely by persons with wheat sensitivity. You can also find low sodium whole grain bread for those restricting sodium intake. Rye breads are always popular, especially those made with a sourdough culture, but remember that they almost always contain wheat gluten, which is the crux of many allergies.

Practically every shape and type of bread that was formerly only available in a white flour and sugar version is now on the shelves of natural food stores made with whole wheat and honey: English muffins, bagels, dinner rolls, hot dog and hamburger buns, French bread, even pizza crusts and pie shells.

A few breads may be new to many people, for although some of them have been around for thousands of years they are relatively recent transplants to the American culture. *Pita* bread, sometimes called *pocket* bread or *Bible Bread*, is enjoying a Western revival due to renewed interest in Middle Eastern foods. This round flat bread, usually made from whole wheat flour, water, yeast, and salt, can be opened up to form a pocket which may be stuffed with whatever you want. The traditional stuffing is falafel and hummous, but tofu or avocado seem to wind up inside just as often. Supermarkets may carry a white flour version of pita bread so be sure to check your labels.

Unleavened breads, or flatbreads, made solely from whole grains and water, without any leavening agents, have now become firmly entrenched in the natural foods movement. From Mexico we have the *tortilla*, traditionally made from stone ground corn and water, sometimes with a trace of lime (the kind that comes from the ground not from trees). The mixture is pressed out into a flat circle about ⅛-inch thick and fried in oil, baked in the oven, or even baked on a rock in the sun if you really want to get back to it all. *Chapatti*, the traditional peasant bread of India, is pretty much the same, except it's made from whole wheat and is usually larger. Both these flatbreads can be eaten by themselves or stuffed and rolled up. Tortillas baked and cut into quarters make great salt-free and fat-free chips for dips.

One of the most interesting breads to arrive on the scene recently is made from a single ingredient. *Sproutbread*, commercially called Essene Bread or Wayfarer's Bread, is a thick mound of sprouted wheat berries put through a course grinder and baked at fairly low temperatures. No yeast is used; no oil, sweetener, nor salt is added. The bread has a chewy consistency and derives is natural sweetness from the sprouted wheat and from a process known as dextrinization, whereby low, slow heat breaks down starches into simple sugars. It isn't the type of bread you would use for a sandwich but is great for eating along with salad or for spreading things on. After the initial success of plain sproutbread, a number of variations appeared and you may now find sproutbread with raisins, seeds, and various fruits and nuts; even one made from sprouted rye berries. Because of its high moisture content, sproutbread molds easily at room temperature and should always be kept frozen or refrigerated.

One of the reasons behind the increasing popularity of pita bread, tortillas, chapattis, and sproutbread is their low calorie value. It is the oil and sweetener that really boost up the calories in bread, not the grain itself. Also, many people who are realizing the value of low oil, low fat diets, and those wishing to avoid all sweeteners and salt, are turning to these products.

Cookies and Cakes

Since the time the first prehistoric man stood up on his hind limbs and raided a bee hive, the sweet tooth has ruled the human psyche. Only those who have never had access or exposure to sweets exist without sugar cravings. And once these people, no matter how primitive or isolated, get their first taste of Coca Cola or Hershey's chocolate, they are forever hooked. Even monkeys, taken straight from the wild, can be turned into sugar addicts in a month, ignoring all their instincts and refusing wholesome food in favor of candy. Those of us who have fought the battle to give up sugar and won, only to succumb to the lure of honey, molasses, and maple syrup, know in their hearts they've only traded one drug for another. Even the chosen few who are able to give up all refined sweets indulge their primitive desires with dates, raisins, and dried figs. True, some do manage to give it all up, but these are special people.

If we admit, then, that we must deal with this monster from

time to time, we ought to at least deal with it in the healthiest way possible. Although no sweet is "good" for you, some are certainly better than others, or at least not as bad. We think the body can tolerate a certain percentage of its daily calories in the form of sugars, and if it's not overdone, there is probably no great harm to the system. Most people committed to a natural diet have therefore accepted that sweets made from whole wheat and honey and other natural ingredients, used sparingly, have their place in a healthy diet. Even if you doubt this deep inside, which I do, reality must be faced, and if you're going to succumb to your sweet tooth occasionally, better with a wholesome carrot cake than sugar-glazed jelly doughnuts.

Not surprisingly, this line of thinking has not been overlooked by the health food industry. Cookies and cakes, ranging in quality from excellent to poor, abound in health and natural food stores. Some stores in fact appear to do the bulk of their business in sweets and vitamin pills. No store, however, could survive very long without something to satiate the universal sweet tooth.

Your two major concerns when selecting cookies and cakes should be freshness and quality of ingredients. Many stores now do their own baking or purchase from local whole grain bakeries, and this gives the consumer greater control of the freshness of the product. Packaged items manufactured and distributed by national companies, however, carry little indication of freshness. Rarely are these products dated, at least in any way the consumer can understand. This does not automatically mean they are stale. Even without chemical preservatives, sound, airtight packaging combined with the natural preservative qualities of honey and other sweeteners will provide most of these products with a reasonable shelf life. Again, the store that buys in small quantities and turns over its inventory is your best bet.

The basic ingredients you want to look for in your bakery snack are whole wheat flour, a natural sweetener, a nonhydrogenated oil, like soy, corn, safflower, or no oil, and natural flavors and colors. Try to avoid the white sugar-white flour syndrome and the hydrogenated oils. Not all cookies and cakes found in natural food stores will necessarily conform to these ideals, so read labels carefully. Remember, the retailer, in addition to providing a central place where good food may be purchased, also has to pay the rent. To do that he may carry products that he does not necessarily believe in but that many of his customers nevertheless demand. His only obligation is to see that his products are fairly and correctly labelled; it's up to you to do your homework.

A perfect example is *Tiger's Milk Cookies*, one of the oldest and most popular of the health snacks. You would be hard pressed to find a store without them, yet their ingredients leave much to be desired. Enriched white flour, brown sugar, and hydrogenated or partially hydrogenated soy and palm oils all rank high in the hierarchy of ingredients. Whole wheat fig bars from *Famous Foods of Virginia* is another. Granted Famous Foods uses figs and whole wheat flour, but that's about the only redeeming feature in a product otherwise filled with brown sugar, corn syrup, white sugar, dextrose, partially hydrogenated oils, and even artificial color.

This is not to say you won't find good products made with wholesome ingredients, only that you should read labels and not make any assumptions.

Crackers and Chips

The same precautions that we applied to breads, cakes, and cookies apply to crackers and chips. A check of the ingredients list may reveal you're not getting what you expected. Famous Foods of Virginia markets several types of popular and inexpensive crackers: Stoned Wheat Wafers, Sesame Crisps, and Roman Meal Crackers, all of which are made with white flour and vegetable shortening. What is vegetable shortening? I'm always a little skeptical when I see that on a label; it's just not specific enough. After all, Crisco is vegetable shortening, and I don't think I'd care to eat a lot of that. It seems that if they were using good quality oil they would be happy to state that on the label. Better, although blander, are rice cakes by Chico San or Arden to name only two. These are pressed from puffed brown rice and come in salted and unsalted versions. They don't contain many nutrients, due to the heat involved in the puffing process, but they are at least made from whole grains. Rice cakes are good for people who want to avoid oils in particular.

As you might expect, virtually any cracker you find in a supermarket made from refined products has its whole grain counterpart available in natural food stores. I've even seen whole wheat Matzohs.

"Healthy" chips differ from regular chips only in the type of oil used and the absence of preservatives like BHT. Whether any potato chip can rightfully be called "healthy" is questionable, since the oil content is so high. The total amount of fat in a potato chip is *120 times* the amount found in the slice of potato it was made from. Health food chips will of course be made with safflower or corn oil as opposed to the hydrogenated lard often used in commercial chips, but it's still fat. Chips also contain a lot of salt, so keep that in mind when you start munching down a bag or two. Many companies now offer salt-free versions of all their chips.

Because of their high oil content, chips can go rancid quickly. Some companies clearly mark their products with expiration dates, but many do not, or if they do it is in some kind of code unfathomable to the buying public. All things considered, chips do not stack up as a quality food, but if that type of snack is important to you, you're somewhat better off with a natural food brand than the mass-market type.

Pasta

Pasta, of course, is the general term for all forms of spaghetti, macaroni, lasagne, noodles, and so forth. Virtually every size and shape available in the supermarket made from refined semolina flour is sold in natural food stores in a whole grain version. The wheat often used is durum wheat, a grain so hard that bread made from it would be suitable for building a patio. This very quality makes it perfect for pasta, since it will stay together while being cooked in a variety of ways.

Whole wheat pasta is an excellent food, since it contains all the goodness of whole grains and lots of slow-burning complex carbohydrates for energy production. Its real value, however, is its versatility. Pasta opens up so many new creative possibilities in a grain-centered diet often limited by the blandness of rice and potatoes.

Durum wheat is almost always the base of any whole grain pasta, although lots of other grains and vegetable powders are added for variety. A natural food store with space enough to offer a wide range of pasta will have available soy pasta, sesame pasta, spinach pasta, and artichoke pasta, as well as straight whole wheat pasta. All of these contain whole wheat with the addition of dehydrated spinach powder, soy flour, or sesame seed powder, etc. Also, other grains may be added to produce soy-rice pasta, corn pasta, buckwheat pasta, and so forth. One of the most popular is the colorful vegetable elbows made from durum wheat and a number of dehydrated vegetable powders: spinach, artichoke, carrot, and others. Spaghetti, elbows, fettuccini noodles, lasagne noodles, stuffing shells, spirals, wheels, and even alphabets are available.

Pasta is probably one of the easiest ways to introduce whole grains to a family trying to break the refined food habit. Green spaghetti or brightly colored vegetable elbows are enough of a novelty to get kids to at least try them. The texture is a bit coarser than white flour pasta, but one adjusts to it quickly.

Preparation of whole grain pasta is the same as refined pasta, although cooking times may be a bit longer. Just throw your pasta into boiling water, salted to taste if you wish, and boil until tender. This generally takes about 15 minutes, but taste is always the best guide. Pasta that is going to be baked after boiling, like lasagne noodles or stuffing shells, is best not fully cooked in the water, since it will continue to soften in the oven.

The density and low oil and moisture content of durum wheat gives it a long shelf life, so spoilage is not the problem it is with bread. Pasta remains stable for long periods if stored under reasonable conditions. Hot, moist places are to be avoided since they can promote molding.

Some companies, like Westbrae, are now making their pasta exclusively from organically grown wheat. This is a welcome sight on the shelves and the cost difference is slight.

Recipes

Basic Whole Wheat Bread[5]

2½ cups warm water (110°–115°F)
6–8 cups whole wheat flour
2 Tbsp. active dry yeast

Pour warm water into large bowl. Sprinkle yeast on top of water. After about 3 minutes the yeast will bubble to the top. Then stir in half of the flour and beat well, until dough becomes smooth (100 strokes). Cover; let rise about 1½ hours. Add the remaining flour, one cup at a time, mixing well after each cup.

Knead in the bowl until dough does not stick to bowl, then turn out onto a floured board. Flour your hands. Knead, push and fold, adding flour as necessary to prevent the dough from sticking to the board. Continue kneading until dough is soft and springy and does not stick to hands or board. Return to bowl. Cover with a damp towel and set in a warm place. Allow to rise until double in bulk. Divide dough in half, shape into oblongs and place into two well oiled loaf pans. (Sprinkle with cornmeal to make removing easier). Cover and let rise until doubled. Place in preheated oven and bake for 50 minutes at 325°.

Low-Fat Bran Muffins[8]

2 cups whole wheat pastry flour
2 cups bran
1 tsp. baking soda
½ tsp. baking powder
2 egg whites
2 cups nonfat buttermilk or skim milk
½ cup undiluted frozen apple juice concentrate, thawed
½ tsp. cinnamon
⅛ tsp. cloves
⅛ tsp. nutmeg
½ tsp. vanilla

Sift together the dry ingredients, except the bran, in a mixing bowl. Now mix in the bran. Beat the egg whites until stiff peaks form. Add the liquid ingredients to the dry ingredients, folding in the egg whites last. Bake 20 minutes in nonstick muffin tins in a preheated, 400°F oven.

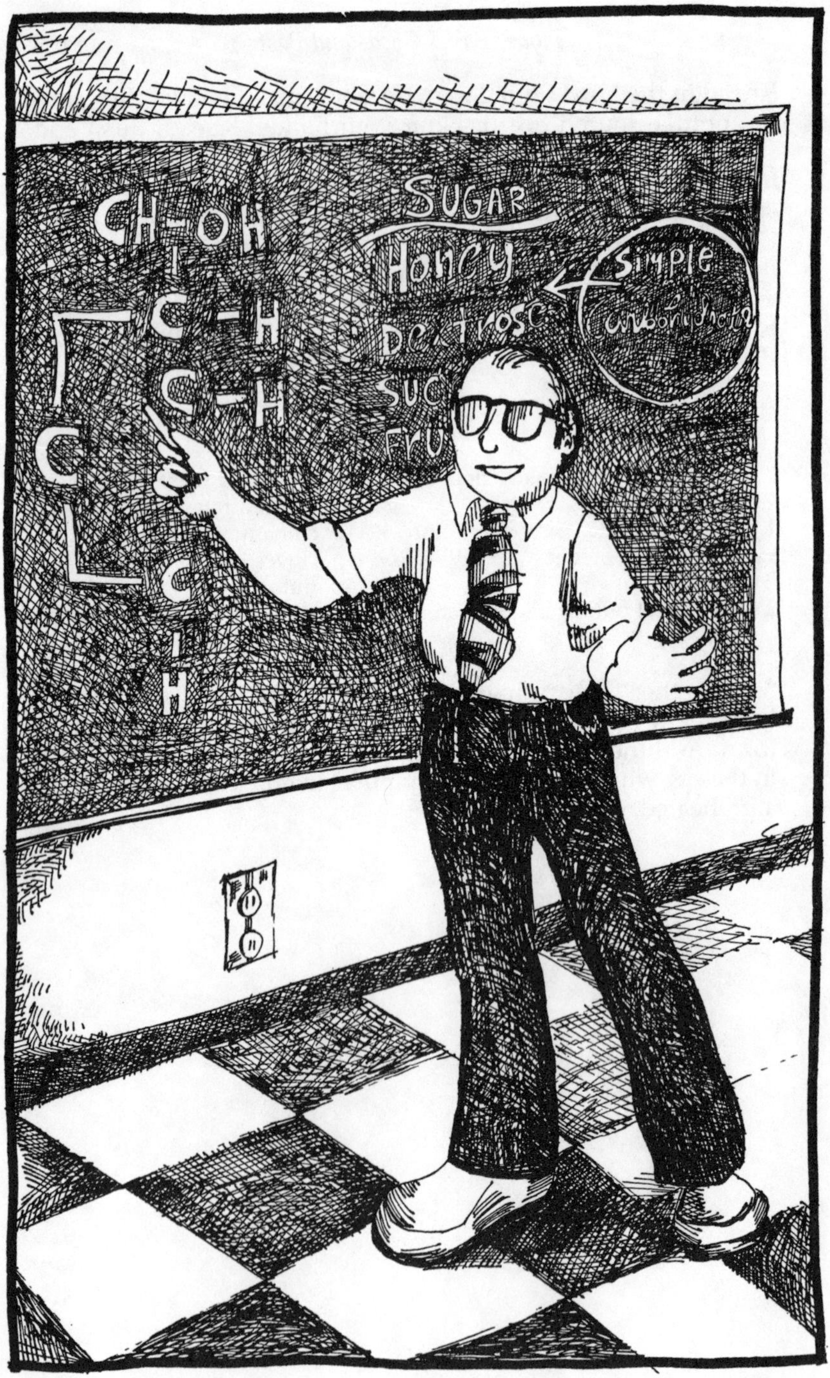
CH-OH
C-H
C-H
SUGAR
Honey
Dextrose
simple

CHAPTER 10

Sweeteners

I have to assume that anyone who has bothered to read this far already knows that white sugar is not a natural food and not desirable in a healthy diet, although they may not necessarily know why. As we look at the sugar problem and discuss alternative sweeteners, I hope to induce you to consider the dubious value of all concentrated sweeteners, even that paragon of Nature's creations, honey.

White Sugar

Sugar cane and sugar beets, the two most common sources of refined sugar, are both natural foods. They contain fiber, vitamins, minerals, amino acids, and trace elements, in every way conforming to our definition of natural foods. Where people consume sugar cane directly, they take in far less sugar than Americans do and do not develop as much sugar-related disease. Once again, Nature understands the importance of the balance among nutrients in a food, and this balance is protective. It is only when Man, through technology, chooses to *isolate* one component out of this natural balance of nutrients that the trouble begins. The natural buffering action of fiber is lost, the nutrients which aid digestion are lost, and the isolated substance behaves like a totally different animal, in this case a nasty one.

The refinement process strips the sugar cane or beet step by step until all that remains is one substance, called sucrose, which consists of two simple sugars, glucose and fructose. Glucose is absorbed in the intestine, and travels to the liver, where most of it is metabolized for energy. A small amount is stored as glycogen in the liver and muscle tissue for use in future energy requiring activities. Any excess is converted to fat and stored, except for very small amounts that undergo biochemical conversions for necessary body functions. Fructose is converted into glucose by the liver and stored as fat if it is not needed for energy.

So what does all this mean? After all, every carbohydrate is eventually broken down into glucose, so what's the big deal about white sugar? First, since refined sugar contains no fiber, it is absorbed too rapidly into the system. This induces certain organs, like the pancreas and adrenal glands, to overreact each time refined sugar is ingested. It is thought that continuous demands of this nature upon these glands causes eventual damage to them. Second, the lack of vitamins and minerals in refined sugar makes it a "nutrient thief" so to speak, that is, it steals nutrients from the body for its digestion but supplys none of its own.[1] Sugar has been accused of consisting of "empty calories," a fair description by any yardstick. Third, refined sugar tends to inhibit the ability of white blood cells to surround invading germs, thus increasing the individual's susceptibility to disease. A person consuming sugar on a regular basis could expect lowered resistance to bacteria.

The facts and theories surrounding sugar's relationship to human disease are very controversial. It is difficult to experiment with human beings, and laboratory animals are not always the most reliable indicators of what's going on in the human system. People's diets are complex, and those eating large amounts of refined sugar are almost always eating large amounts of fats, and probably a good share of chemical additives as well, so it is hard to separate the possible causes of a manifested disease. Some say sugar is the prime cause of heart disease; others say cholesterol, fat, or even basic vitamin and mineral imbalances are the culprits. A person eating a junk food diet has all the above going for him. It's hard to miss when you've covered all the bases. The best defense obviously is to try to eliminate as many of these potential causes of degenerative disease as we can without making our lives unbearably boring.

Alternative Sweeteners

As you browse through any natural foods cookbook you will find a fairly wide assortment of sweeteners recommended as replacements for white sugar. Although none of these will be as inexpensive as white sugar, the extra cost is not usually that great, especially if you start thinking of sweets as special foods which you allow yourself to indulge in only occasionally, rather than as a regular part of your daily diet.

Raw Sugar (Turbinado Sugar)

The term "raw sugar" is unfortunate. It gives the impression to the consumer that he is buying some sort of raw, unprocessed agricultural product, like whole sugar cane ground up into a useable form. In actuality, the raw sugar you purchase in natural food stores is for the most part a highly refined product, having gone through all the same refinement stages as white sugar except for the final extraction of molasses. If white sugar is 99 percent refined, then raw sugar is 95 percent refined. To say that raw sugar is better for you than white sugar is like saying that 90 proof vodka won't harm you as much as 100 proof vodka. Technically, both statements may be correct, but from the practical point of view there's really no difference.

Brown Sugar (Yellow-D Sugar)

Brown sugar is white sugar with the molasses added back into it. Generally more molasses is added back than was taken out, the result being that brown sugar usually contains a good deal more nutrients than raw sugar, which supposedly has not had the molasses completely removed. This is not to say that brown sugar is therefore a nutritious food; it is not. It may contain small amounts of calcium, iron, and potassium, but it is still 93.8 percent pure carbohydrate (white sugar is 99.9 percent), and is still a highly refined product with no fiber and no B vitamins.

Fructose

Fructose is often referred to as fruit sugar, since it is commonly found in fruit. The fructose you buy in the store, however, is a refined product which has probably never seen a fruit, being derived from beets or corn. You will recall that sucrose (white sugar) consists of glucose and fructose. To produce isolated fructose the sucrose compound in white sugar is cut in half, leaving glucose and fructose as separate entities. Fructose has no nutritional value except for calories in the form of pure carbohydrate. What accounts for the popularity of fructose is the fact that it does not involve insulin from the pancreas for its assimilation in the body and thus represents a "safer" sugar for diabetics. This is misleading, however, since diabetics may use it only in small amounts, and it becomes nothing more than another "exchange" on their restricted diets. Diabetics would do much better to use up their daily sugar allotment by eating whole fresh fruit and steering away from products sweetened with fructose.

Remember also that it is the fructose part of sucrose that is converted so readily to fat. Consuming too much fructose may lead to elevated triglyceride (fat) levels in the bloodstream, and there is much evidence to suggest that this state is a prime cause of atherosclerosis or hardening of the arteries. This should not be interpreted to mean that eating fruit will lead to the same state—it will not. As always, Nature has designed her products carefully, and the balance of fruits' fiber and nutrients protects us from overconsumption of fructose.

Fructose gained its popularity mostly as the result of a fad diet which used it in granulated or tablet form to curb the appetite by maintaining high blood sugar levels all day. This is not a very sensible way to diet. The waxing and waning of blood sugar levels is a natural body process and should be aided and abetted by a whole food diet, which accomplishes this change gently. Fad diets are designed largely to sell books and make a few people rich.

Date Sugar

Dates have an abundance of natural sugar, probably the highest of any fruit, making them an ideal, although expensive, sweetener. Date sugar is produced by dehydrating and grinding up pitted dates, producing a fairly coarse brown meal with a distinct flavor. Since it is as close to a whole food as one can get in a powdered sweetener, it is fairly nutritious. Unfortunately, date sugar tends to ferment easily; often chemical preservatives are added to extend the life of the product, or compounds like sodium silico aluminate are added as anticaking agents. Pure date sugar without additives is available, however.

Molasses

A major step in refining sugar from cane is the extraction of molasses. Actually this occurs at several stages in the process. The initial separation of syrup from crystals, accomplished by a centrifuge, results in a fairly good quality molasses, with substantial amounts of calcium, iron, potassium, and small amounts of B vitamins. Toward the end of the process, while the sugar is still "raw," a final extraction is made which produces a low grade weakened syrup known as *blackstrap molasses*. Blackstrap, though long heralded in health food circles for its miraculous powers, possesses no magic but does contain considerably larger amounts of minerals and slightly larger amounts of vitamins than first extraction molasses. The sugar content of molasses ranges from 55 percent for blackstrap to 65 percent for first extraction syrup.

Malt Syrup

If barley is allowed to sprout, it develops diastase enzymes, which possess the ability to change starches into sugars. If this *diastatic malt*, as it is now called, is added to a starch (like cornstarch), fermentation takes place which produces either malt syrup or malt sugar, depending upon how soon the drying process is halted. The resulting syrup is a unique tasting sweetener, with some iron and a few B vitamins, but largely consisting of maltose and dextrin.

Sorghum Syrup

Derived from the stalks of sorghum plants, sorghum syrup or sorghum "molasses," as it is sometimes called, is not common in the commercial marketplace. It has a taste similar to cane molasses and possesses a few minerals like iron and calcium, but like all sweeteners, it is largely sugar—sucrose in this case.

Rice Syrup

The increasing Japanese influence in the natural foods market has introduced us to rice syrup, a sweetener produced by the same technique as malt syrup, using rice starch instead of corn. I have not come across a nutritional analysis of rice syrup, but I imagine it to be comparable to malt or sorghum.

Maple Syrup

When one thinks of maple syrup, two pictures come to mind. The first is a stack of steaming hot, nutritious pancakes and the second is a Vermont farmer in bib overalls lovingly collecting this pure amber liquid in a seasoned oak bucket—straight from nature to your breakfast table.

Unfortunately, neither image corresponds to reality these days. Most pancakes come from packaged, add-water-and-stir preparations consisting largely of white flour, and good old pure maple syrup simply ain't what it used to be.

Although I have no doubt there are still plenty of small, independent, maple syrup producers collecting the tree sap, the chances are pretty strong that you will never see any of this unless you visit them personally. Maple syrup today is collected by "modern" methods, emphasizing, as usual, efficiency and profit over quality. When the maple tree is tapped it attempts to close up this "wound," as any sensible organism would. Since this would impede the flow of sap, a formaldehyde pellet is plugged into the tap-hole to prevent closure. Next, a tap is put in and the sap runs past the formaldehyde pellet through polyvinylchloride tubing to a main collector. Do you think any of that formaldehyde is getting into the syrup? And what about the tubing? Polyvinylchloride (PVC) is notorious for its instability, particularly in the presence of heat (the sun, for example). Think any plastic is getting into your maple syrup? Hmmm.

The next step is to change the colorless liquid coming out of the tree into that rich brown nectar flowing over the top of your waffles. This is accomplished by heating the sap at high temperatures across metal sheets until it turns brown, a process known as caramelizing.

As if that's not enough, it may also be strained through cloth mesh which has been routinely bleached with sodium hypochlorite to prevent mold formation.

So, this originally colorless liquid, consisting of 98 percent water and 2 percent sucrose (white sugar), is now a brown caramelized syrup possibly laced with formaldehyde, PVC, and sodium hypochlorite, and appearing on your breakfast table in a down home-style, tin can labeled "Pure Maple Syrup." Spare me.

By the way, the maple syrup I'm describing is the stuff sold in natural food stores. The supermarket brands, which are usually just called "pancake syrup," are made of corn syrup and sugar syrup with perhaps 2 percent maple syrup added, or even just artificial maple flavor.

Canadian maple syrup producers do not routinely use formaldehyde pellets, and if you can locate a brand from Canada you will at least be spared that particular excipient.

Contrary to what is often believed, maple syrup contains little in the way of nutrients other than carbohydrate. It is 98 percent sugar and water with a sprinkling of minerals, and no vitamins to speak of.

Honey

Along with whole wheat flour, honey is one of the key foods automatically associated with the change away from unnatural processed foods. In many ways, however, honey is a processed food, refined by bees instead of Man. As the worker bee makes her daily rounds in the neighborhood, she extracts nectar from the various local flowers and stores it in a special honey sac to transport it back to the hive, where it is hoarded in combs for future use as a source of carbohydrate energy. Nectar, one component of the whole flower, consists almost entirely of pure carbohydrate, specifically a mixture of glucose and fructose. There is no fiber and only insignificant traces of vitamins and minerals. The pure nectar is a highly refined food. If Man were to make honey without bees he would probably collect millions of flowers, boil them down, and centrifuge out the nectar much the same way molasses is extracted from sugar cane. Bees accomplish this task far more efficiently, however, and Man needs only collect the fruits of their labor.

As bees gather nectar, they also collect a rather remarkable substance called pollen. Pollen is a powerhouse of nutrients and is mixed with the honey and stored as a source of protein, vitamins, and minerals for the bee colony. If you were to eat honey directly from the hive with its share of pollen (and beeswax), you would be eating a much improved food—still a refined food, and still one to be eaten sparingly, but definitely in a different class than other sweeteners. Unfortunately honey is practically never available in this crude form, at least not commercially.

Treatment of the honey from this point on varies with the producer. In most cases the honey is heated to 150° F or more in order to make it flow more easily and to inhibit granulation or "hardening," and filtered to remove impurities, producing a crystal clear syrup. Ironically, the "impurities" removed through filtration are pollen and beeswax, the two substances that would give the honey a decent measure of nutritional value. And 150° heat readily destroys all of the live enzymes and natural antibiotic properties inherent to raw honey. What remains then is a sugar syrup, clear and attractive, but not quite what the bees had in mind.

But wait a second! That honey I bought yesterday at the health food store clearly stated on the label: "Raw, Organic, Uncooked, Unfiltered, Natural Honey." Did I miss something? Yes, because what wasn't on the label and should have been is a little asterisk next to each word and a footnote saying "this term has no legal definition and is therefore meaningless." "Organic" means nothing since bees obviously don't collect nectar from plastic flowers. The law does not consider 150° to be cooking, so the honey may still be called raw and uncooked although most of the good stuff has been destroyed by heat. As for filtering, any honey clear enough to see through has been filtered regardless of what the label states. True unfiltered honey is murky and clouded with pollen particles and wax.

Don't despair. It is possible to obtain good quality honey from small local sources; you just have to take the time to check them out. Often natural food stores and co-ops buy directly from private beekeepers who work *with* instead of against the bees and aren't inclined to process their honey. They usually have a settling tank, so the honey may not contain all the usual "impurities," but you'll still be getting a better deal than you would by buying a national brand. If you have no local source, check out the popular brands for the best buy. Forget about the raw, organic business, but look for the word "unheated," not "uncooked," on the label. This is supposed to mean that no heat has ever been applied. Also check the clarity of the honey and go for the ones you can't see through. The U.S. Dept. of Agriculture grades honey according to its clarity, which of course is a reflection of how much it is filtered. In typical government fashion, the honeys with the greatest clarity receive the highest grades. Grade "A" or "Fancy" honey has been screened and filtered to death. Lower grades are B (Choice), C (Standard), and D (Substandard). These grades imply nothing about the quality of the honey or its source, but only indicate the degree of fineness of the screen through which the honey has been filtered.

Some stores carry a dazzling array of varietal honeys: sage honey, orange honey, clover honey, desert flower honey, buckwheat honey, alfalfa honey, eucalyptus honey, and so on. These names supposedly refer to the flowers prevalent in the area surrounding the hives from which the honey was extracted, but I have heard from reputable sources that a number of major companies draw many of their varieties from the same vat and just randomly slap on different labels. Besides, like wine, a honey does not legally have to be exclusively from a single source in order to be labeled as such. Many states require only 51 percent to be from the labeled source, the balance being just about anything. Not that any of this makes much difference once the honey has been heated and filtered, despite wild claims often made about the superiority of one honey over another.

When it comes to taste, however, honeys are definitely different, and there are honey aficionados just as there are wine aficionados. Honeys range in taste from mild sweetness similar to sugar and water to a biting, even burning harshness.

Consistency also varies from free-flowing syrup to honey so hard you need a knife to cut it. The differences are mainly due to glucose content—the higher, the more inclined the honey is to granulate, although all honeys will granulate eventually if unheated and allowed to sit long enough in cool temperatures. As mentioned, honey producers heat their honey to inhibit granulation and facilitate bottling procedures. But granulation doesn't guarantee that a honey has not been heated, since dry honey crystals may be added to induce granulation in the bottle.

You will occasionally see "comb honey" for sale, and if you can verify that it has been taken directly from the hive it is an excellent purchase, since it is as close to the source as possible. The comb itself is made of beeswax and may be chewed like gum.

As always, seeing should not necessarily be believing. Honey in a comb is no guarantee of purity. Some producers cook and filter their honey and then pour it into a jar with a clean comb. Nothing is sacred.

You may be interested to know that although honey has little nutritional value and is almost exclusively used as a pleasure food, much folklore and some scientific evidence attest to its medicinal value. Honey has been used quite successfully to treat "local allergies," that is, allergies to pollen in the air often developed by people migrating to a new locality. The pollens in the honey, like vaccines, induce the production of antibodies to combat the allergy. Real raw honey has genuine bacteria fighting abilities when applied to wounds, and honey's hydroscopic nature (the tendency to absorb moisture from the air) makes it useful for burns where intense local dehydration is a prime enemy. Stories about honey's positive effects on heart problems, arthritis, and even aging abound, although none of this has been scientifically proven. Pollen, as we shall see later, is quite a different story, and it is conceivable that many of the powers attributed to honey are found in the pollen consumed in crude honey.

For most of us, of course, honey will remain a sweetener only, and despite its non-nutritive status, it still makes us feel a lot better to use something more natural than white sugar. Baking with honey takes a bit of getting used to. Honey will alter the taste and, since it is liquid, the texture of baked goods. When substituting honey in recipes calling for any kind of dry sugar, you may use up to 50 percent less honey, since the fructose part of it has a sweeter taste, and you should reduce any liquids in the recipe somewhat since honey obviously contains water. Recipes calling for honey take all of this into account, but if you're devising your own or making natural food substitutions in an old favorite recipe, a little trial and error experimentation may be necessary.

Finally, a word about storage. Honey is its own preservative, and bacteria simply cannot live in something that sweet, so refrigeration is not necessary. In fact, storing it in a warm place is best since it will maintain its pourable consistency. If it granulates and you'd rather it didn't, place the jar in hot water for a short time and it will liquify. The only enemy of honey is moisture. Keep honey in as dry a place as possible, avoiding damp cellars and the like, and keep a tight lid on it. Remember it has the distinct property of extracting moisture from the air around it and this moisture will ultimately cause it to ferment.

Are Sweeteners Natural Foods?

By our definition, or anyone else's for that matter, it would be difficult to classify any of these sweeteners as natural foods. Raw sugar, brown sugar, maple syrup, and the rest have been so refined and isolated from their original sources and are so deficient in the essential nutrients common to these sources that one would be hard pressed to find benefits to the human body. Add to this what we know of sweeteners' negative side effects, including their excessive demands upon the pancreas and their use of stored nutrients for digestion, and their value appears even more dubious. Even honey, regarded by many as the perfect natural food, is a refined and isolated set of sugars, with little nutritional benefit except as a source of quick energy for athletes or for elderly people with severe digestive difficulties.

If these sweeteners are not natural foods, should they all be excluded from the true natural foods diet? I'm afraid the answer is yes, or at least that is the goal we should be working toward. Whether or not we ever achieve it completely is a problem we must each deal with in our own way, but steps ought to be taken in that direction. With the exception of a little iron here and a little calcium there, no sweetener has much nutritional value. They are all "empty calories" in a sense, just like white sugar, and they all replace foods which would offer better nutrition.

This is of course the ideal, perhaps to be admired rather than achieved. Yet the statistics tell us that each and every living American consumes 1 pound of sugar every three days, or 129 pounds a year. Since that includes newborn infants, the elderly, and people who don't consume any at all, those who are eating sugar are no doubt eating considerably more than that. A typical teenager may be taking 40 percent of his calories in the form of sugar. Now, once you've got a raging sweet tooth like this going, switching over to natural foods will help, but not if you simply substitute one sweetener for another. The point is that honey, molasses, and raw sugar usage has to be curtailed severely if we are to achieve healthy minds and bodies. A person eating a diet centering on whole foods can probably afford say 10 percent of his calories in the form of otherwise non-nutritive sweeteners without any great trauma to the body, although he would no doubt be better off without any. Now, 10 percent of a 2500-calorie-a-day diet is about four tablespoons of honey—not at all difficult to come by. A little granola in the morning, some honeyed yogurt at lunch, maybe a sweet dessert and honey in your tea, and you're way over the line. As you can see, getting your sweets intake down to a sensible level will take some careful management.

Beating the Sweet Tooth

The sweet tooth is a monster. We joke about it, we laugh about it, we kid each other about it, but inside we all know it's a monster. It's the monster that brings us tooth decay, obesity, hypoglycemia, and perhaps much more we don't yet know about. Anyone who has gone on a sweet tooth "binge" knows how it can get hold of you and almost control you for periods of time. But the sweet tooth can be managed, controlled, subdued, even beaten. You may never totally eliminate sweets from your life as some have, but you can learn to enjoy an occasional treat or reward without becoming obsessed with more.

What is the sweet tooth? If we're going to beat it we ought to understand what we're fighting. I know of no accepted definition of the sweet tooth other than something vague like "intense craving for sweets . . ." which is not very helpful. First, the sweet tooth is a habit, right? Right. And habits develop due to reinforcement, or reward. In other words if we do something and we are rewarded for it in some way, we are more likely to do it again, providing the reward was positive. So what's the reward for eating something sweet? We could say it's the taste, but that doesn't really hold up. Lots of things taste good. Pizza tastes good, but you don't see millions of people running around with a pizza tooth. Apples taste good, peanut butter tastes good, lots of things taste good.

Now, food gives us energy, right? Right. And energy is definitely a positive reward. Sweets give us energy, so do potatoes. The big difference is that sweets give us energy almost immediately but potatoes do so slowly and steadily. The energy from potatoes is released as they are gradually digested, maintaining a constant and conservative level of blood sugar, which translates into energy, but refined sweeteners enter the bloodstream quickly and give us a "rush" of energy. Not only is this a positive reward but it occurs so close in time to the ingestion of the sugar that we have no doubt what caused it. The unconscious mind makes a definite connection between the cause and the effect. Just like a laboratory rat who presses the right lever and gets a pellet of food, we are likely to repeat an act that gives us immediate satisfaction.

If we accept the sweet tooth as a learned habit, a conditioned response, we can perhaps deal with it on a practical level. Going "cold turkey" is not the answer. Breaking strong habits by stopping them abruptly often causes great stress or the development of new habits that may be worse. One way to work on it might be by *reducing the intensity of the reward*. In other words, if the energy surge we receive from a sweet food is lessened in magnitude, the reward is not as great, and the tendency to repeat the action is somewhat lessened. So, if we design a little program for ourselves in which we gradually reduce the reward by manipulating the quality and quantity of sweetener in our foods, we may be able to bring the monster under control.

Some of the sweeteners discussed earlier may be helpful at the beginning of this program. One of the problems with white sugar is that it has no taste other than just "sweet"; we tend, therefore, to overuse it, since foods are rarely considered "too sweet." Molasses, malt syrup, sorghum, and many grades of honey, on the other hand, have distinct flavors which tend to limit their usage. In other words, too much molasses or too much honey is obvious, since the taste of whatever you're putting it in will become unpleasantly dominated by that particular sweetener. So, just by substituting molasses or honey for sugar you can reduce the amount of total sweetener and also the amount of "instant energy" rushing into your bloodstream. If our "habit theory" is correct, the reward will be less and so will your tendency to repeat the act, i.e., eat more sweets.

The next step, and this will only work if you're preparing your own sweets, is to reduce the amount of sweetener in your recipes. You will be amazed how much you can cut the honey in a cookie or cake recipe without consciously noticing the lessening of sweetness. This may be done gradually so that you and whoever else you are trying to wean from sugar will never notice the changes.

A major move forward is to discontinue using all conventional sweeteners and begin using only fruits and fruit juices in your recipes. Fruits like raisins and dates may be cooked down and blended into syrups which will contain much of their original fiber and most of the nutrients, except those few destroyed by cooking. The sugars contained in these syrups do not rush into the system as rapidly as refined sugars and your "rewards" are again decreased. Bananas also make a good sweetener, as does carob powder and any fruit juice or fruit juice concentrate. You can make soft drinks for the kids by mixing any natural fruit juice with a carbonated mineral water. And if you're fortunate enough to have a Champion Juicer you can put peeled frozen bananas through it and produce a treat that's so much like ice cream you can fool anyone, yet it consists of a single ingredient—bananas, as natural a sweet as you can find. In general, using fruits for sweetening will automatically reduce the total amount of sugar and calories you're taking in.

Once you get this far, you may find that you and your family have reduced your sweet cravings to the point where fruit alone is satisfying. You've come a long way, baby. Fruits will give you the energy you want, but in more reasonable doses, and they won't cause harm to your glandular system or rob your body of vitamins. In addition, they will keep your bowels moving freely so that wastes don't accumulate in your lower digestive areas and cause problems.

Before leaving this subject, I should point out one common pitfall that is easy to succumb to in this type of sweet reduction program. Years ago, when the Surgeon General determined that cigarette smoking was hazardous to our health and something called "tar" was indicted as the offender, cigarette manufacturers began marketing "low tar" smokes. So many guilty smokers began using these heavily filtered cigarettes that the competition became intense, and each new brand boasted less and less tar coming through their miracle filters. All this seemed to be a step in the right direction. I mean, if you have to smoke, better to use a cigarette that reduces the intake of hazardous substances, right? Wrong. Not wrong in principle, it's just that it doesn't really work. Recent studies have shown that smokers using low tar cigarettes characteristically take longer draws on their cigarettes, hold the smoke in their lungs longer, and smoke more often. The bottom line is that they are probably getting no less tar than they used to, they just work harder to get it. This probably explains why the major tobacco companies have suffered no loss of profit despite the Surgeon General's mandatory message and the ban on TV advertising, and neither have those who make their living performing lung surgery.

What all this has to do with sweets is simply that when we begin reducing the amount of sweetener in our goodies we must regulate our intake to avoid eating twice as many goodies to make up for the decreased sweetness. You must allot yourself a certain amount of treats and savor them with respect. Use them sparingly, and watch out for binges. It will take a bit of work, but the monster can be beaten.

Recipes

Here are a few dessert recipes that use no traditional refined sweeteners.

Apple Crisp[6]

6 large red delicious apples, peeled and sliced
20 soft dates, cut into pieces

1 cup water or 1 cup pineapple or apple juice

Place apples and dates in baking dish.

Topping:
2 cups quick-cooking oatmeal
1 cup whole wheat pastry flour
½ tsp. salt

½ cup oil
¼ cup water

Mix the above ingredients well. Into a cup mix oil and water with a fork and add to oats and flour. Mix well. Put on top of apple and date mixture.

Bake on bottom rack at 350–375°F for 45 minutes or until done. If topping browns too quickly, lower temperature.

Banana Cream Pie[6]

½ cup raw cashews
    (or blanched almonds)
12 pitted dates
1 tsp. vanilla
2 cups water

½ tsp. salt
Bananas, ripe and speckled, about 2 or 3
strawberries (optional)

Blend all ingredients except bananas in a blender. Place in pan and cook 20 minutes or more, stirring constantly to keep from sticking until it thickens. Cool and place in refrigerator until ready to use. Using your favorite pie crust slice bananas lengthwise and cover bottom of crust, then spoon in a layer of filling, then another layer of bananas, etc., until full. Top with strawberries, if desired.

French Apple Tart[8]

1 cup Grape Nuts cereal
3 Tbsp. undiluted frozen apple juice concentrate, thawed
3 medium apples, cored and thinly sliced

2 tsp. lemon juice
½ tsp. cinnamon

Topping
1 Tbsp. cornstarch
½ cup undiluted frozen apple juice concentrate, thawed

½ cup water

Moisten the cereal with the 3 Tbsp. apple juice concentrate (use a little extra, if needed) and pat the cereal into a thin layer in a nonstick, lined pie pan or ordinary pie pan. Sprinkle with ¼ tsp. cinnamon. Arrange the prepared apple slices in slightly overlapping circles, starting at the outside rim and working toward the center. Sprinkle them with lemon juice and ¼ tsp. cinnamon. Cover with foil and bake in a 350°F oven for 45 minutes, or until the apples are tender. Remove from oven and let cool to room temperature. Combine the cornstarch, ½ cup apple juice concentrate, and water in a saucepan; cook and stir until the mixture thickens and then clears. Spoon or brush this mixture over apples. Chill. Serves 6–8. For added sweetness try adding raisins before baking.

Q. *What do we do when we're invited over to a friend's house for dinner?*

A. Tell your friends to prepare extra vegetables and potatoes for you since you won't be eating much meat (if any). Or, volunteer to bring a dish for everyone—and make it a big pot of brown rice. We've turned many people on to whole grains by bringing a potful for dinner and letting them find out for themselves how much better unprocessed grains taste.

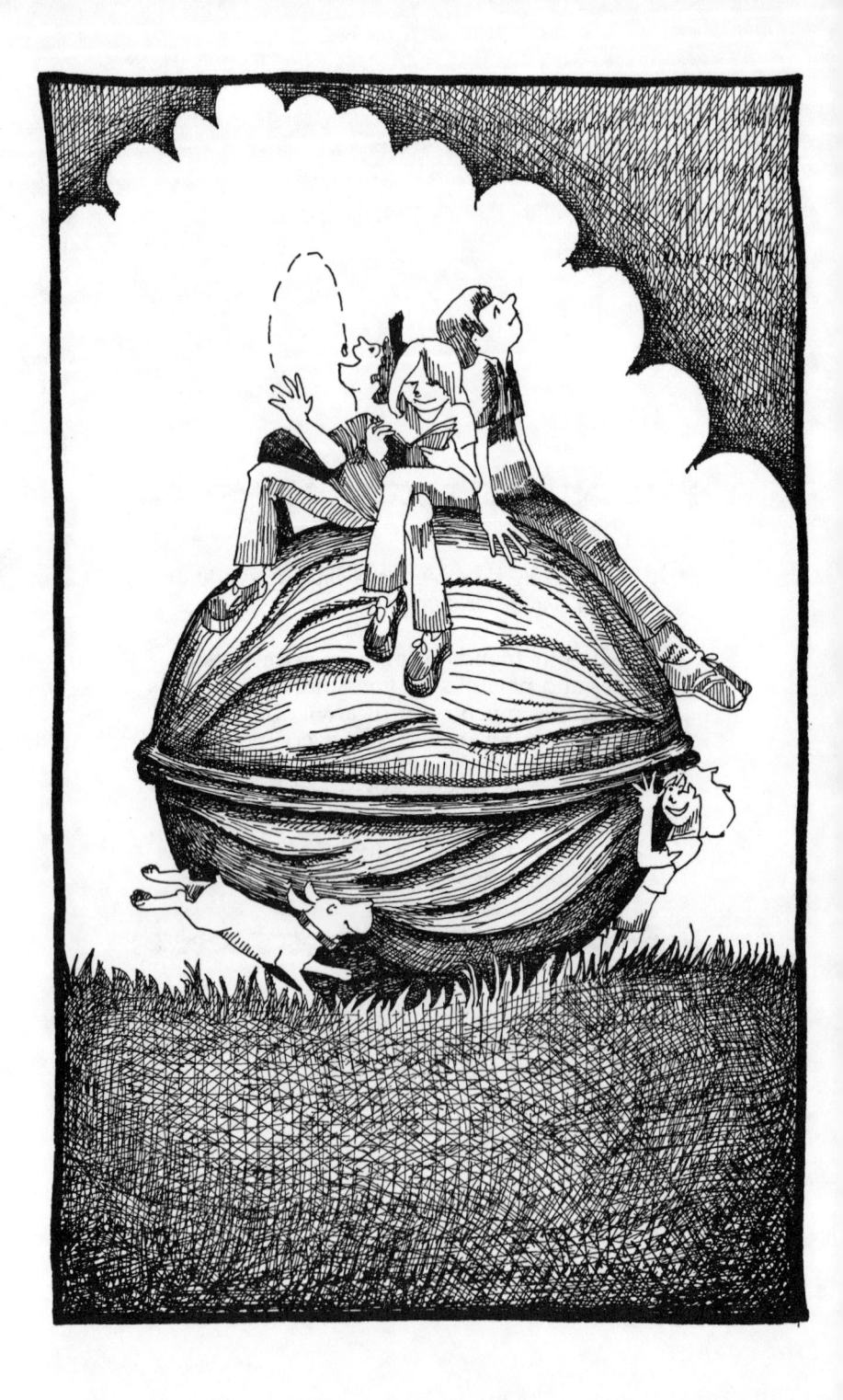

CHAPTER 11

Nuts, Seeds, and Dried Fruits

Ask the average man in the street to draw you a mental picture of a vegetarian, and he will probably describe a thin, pale person hopelessly trying to survive on almonds, raisins, and sunflower seeds. Although it is true that many vegetarians eat a lot of nuts and seeds, the image of them as being in a constant state of imminent malnutrition has long been discredited. In recent years we have seen highly conservative government agencies as well as private medical and scientific organizations admit that the vegetarian diet can be safe and healthy providing the variety of foods is not too severely limited. Textbooks on nutrition and dietetics, which for so long have clung steadfastly to the sacrosanct Four Food Groups, are now talking about "meat, fish, fowl, milk, cheese, and eggs . . ." and adding phrases like ". . . or suitable protein alternatives such as nuts, seeds, legumes. . . ." Of course people have been living long and disease-free lives on these foods for thousands of years, but then they're foreigners and probably don't know any better.

Although nuts and seeds may not be as "perfect" as the egg in terms of amino acid balance, they are nonetheless good sources of complete protein and lack the negative aspects of animal protein, like cholesterol and high concentrations of saturated fat. This is not to say that they are the perfect vegetarian food, since they do have a number of drawbacks. First, the majority of their calories come from oil, largely unsaturated, but often saturated as well. The coconut is an exception, being about 72 percent saturated fat with only a trace of polyunsaturates. The abundance of oil and the lack of water make for digestive difficulties. If nuts and seeds are to be digested and assimilated properly they must be chewed more thoroughly than most people are accustomed to chewing them. Nuts and seeds should become almost liquid in the mouth before swallowing, whereas most of us just break them up a bit and down they go, only to appear intact in the stool a day or so later.

The second problem is the *total* amount of fat. Most enlightened nutritionists these days agree that fats should be carefully controlled in the diet, whether they be saturated animal fats or polyunsaturated vegetable oils. Although the experts disagree on exact figures, most suggest that any more than 20 percent of your daily calories coming from fats and oils exceeds what is healthy. Since most of the popular nuts and seeds range from 45 to 90 percent fat, it is easy to see how moderation is a necessity here.

The third problem is also solved through moderation. Since nuts and seeds are such concentrated foods, a large number of calories are packed into relatively small units. It is very easy to eat too many cashews or pumpkin seeds because they possess so little bulk relative to the amount of calories they add. One cup of peanuts provides over 800 calories, while the same amount of lettuce has 32 calories, strawberries, 55 calories, and cooked brown rice, 178 calories. You would have to eat four and a half cups of brown rice or eight baked potatoes to equal the calories in a single cup of peanuts. The sheer volume of the rice or potatoes makes it all but impossible to consume that many calories in one sitting, while eating a cup of peanuts is a breeze.

All things considered, nuts and seeds are basically fine foods if used sparingly and, preferably, if eaten along with other less concentrated foods. They are high in many important nutrients, including calcium, iron, zinc, vitamin E, and an important constituent of fat, linoleic acid. This is not to say they are essential to a healthy vegetarian diet; they are not. Many vegetarians avoid nuts and seeds entirely for one reason or another and eat perfectly well-balanced diets using only fruits, vegetables, and whole grains. But, if you enjoy nuts and can control your intake, by all means include them in your diet.

As for dried fruits, although they are a concentrated source of calories and should be consumed in moderation, they otherwise present no problems. You should be aware though that certain vitamins, like A and C, are partially or wholly lost during the drying process, and for this reason fresh fruit is always recommended over dried.

Let us now look at each of these three foods, how they are marketed, and how they may best be bought, stored, and consumed for maximum benefit.

Nuts

Besides choosing among the various commonly available nuts, you will also have to choose between shelled and unshelled, raw and roasted, and whole and chopped, slivered, broken, etc. As always there are advantages and disadvantages in each choice.

Shelled or Unshelled?

After most nuts are harvested, the shells are removed by special machinery, and the nut "meats" are packed in bulk containers to be shipped off for direct sale to retail customers or roasting houses, or to be made into a variety of nut products like butters, meals, and oils. Some nuts remain unshelled and are sold this way in retail stores. If natural food stores have the space and demand, they will offer their customers the choice between shelled and unshelled nuts in a number of popular varieties. From a strict nutritional point of view, that is, looking only at an analysis of nutrients, there is no difference. The difference is in freshness and all that implies. Nuts are high in oil, and thus susceptible to rancidity. Of course, the higher the particular nut in oil content, the more likely it is to go rancid. The shell provides a certain degree of natural protection from rancidity. This is not to say a nut will not spoil in the shell, only that the process is retarded considerably by the shell's protective covering. When you remove the shell, the nut meat is exposed to oxygen and the rancidity process begins. Higher fat nuts, like Brazils, macadamias, filberts, pecans, and walnuts, are more vulnerable to spoilage than raw almonds, cashews, and peanuts and should be selected carefully. If you have the choice and don't mind the work, it's always better to buy nuts in the shell and hull them only as you need them. Not only does this more or less guarantee you a fresher, safer product, but it goes a long way toward helping you moderate your intake of nuts. You are far less likely to eat a cup of nuts if you have to crack them by hand.

Roasted or Raw?

Almonds, cashews, peanuts, and pistachios are generally available both raw and roasted. Raw nuts are usually more digestible and nutritious, but the roasted seem to taste better to most people. I highly recommend doing your own roasting, since the roasted nuts you find in natural food stores and elsewhere are often subjected to excessive temperatures and oxygen infiltration in the roasting chamber. The result is significant alterations in the molecular structures of the nut proteins, rendering them relatively indigestible, not to mention the destruction of certain key nutrients. Roasting your own at about 250°F for 50–60 minutes will produce a far better quality product. This does not mean you cannot find safe roasted nuts in the store, you just have to watch the color. The darker the nut as compared to the raw form, the more it has been roasted; the lighter colored nuts are best if you can find them.

Whole or Broken?

Since rancidity is always a problem with nuts, the whole form is preferable to bits, pieces, or slivers. Breaking down whole foods exposes the inner surfaces to the air and increases the rancidity potential geometrically. The smaller the pieces, the higher the risk. Finely ground nut meals and butters, topping the list. Although many people will continue to buy slivered almonds, chopped walnuts, and cashew bits because they are cheaper and more convenient for baking, spending the extra time and money on whole nuts is definitely worth your consideration. As the following list shows, each nut has its individual problems.

Almonds

Almonds grow primarily in the Mediterranean countries and in northern California. You will find them in many forms: in the shell, raw, roasted, bits, slivered, blanched, meal, and butter. They are a good source of protein and important nutrients, but like all nuts are high in fat—although almonds are among the lower oil nuts. In terms of calories they are in the middle range. A cup provides 765 calories.

Like all nuts, almonds may become rancid, although less rapidly than the higher fat nuts like brazils and pecans. Nevertheless, acquiring them in the whole form is always best. Buying in the shell is the ideal way of course, and if you're lucky you can find them with their natural color shell. The bright, pale colored shells found in supermarkets have been bleached with sodium hypochlorite; the natural color is quite a bit darker.

Almonds are graded by the U.S. Dept. of Agriculture on the basis of both quality and size. The highest grades are in the best condition, have the least rancidity, and needless to say are the most expensive. It is probably easiest to judge the quality of almonds visually by noting the number of broken or scarred nuts; the more you see the lower the quality. Don't be deceived by stores selling low priced almonds, which may simply be lower grade nuts.

Occasionally you may chomp into an almond that is distinctly bitter, enough to make you run open-mouthed to the nearest sink or garbage can. Don't worry, you haven't been poisoned. It's just what's known as a "bitter almond," a separate species, perfectly harmless despite its lack of palatability. The highest grades of almonds aren't supposed to have any of these mixed in, but occasionally a few sneak through. If you get more than a few of these bitter fellows in your bag, you've probably purchased a lower grade almond.

Almond meal is occasionally called for in recipes. This is nothing more than ground up almonds, with the consistency of a coarse cornmeal. Although you will find almond meal for sale in some stores, packaged in cans or boxes, I strongly advise you to avoid it, since freshness is dubious. Remember that the more you break down on oil-containing nut, the more you expose it to rancidity. It is also questionable whether any "vacuum packing" technique really precludes this deterioration. If you need almond meal, just throw your almonds into a blender, food processor, nut and seed mill, or an old fashioned, hand meat grinder and use it up immediately, making fresh meal as you need it.

Brazil Nuts

Most of the Brazil nuts I have seen come from Bolivia, where the people probably call them Bolivia nuts. So much for nationalism. The dark, thick shelled nuts you see are actually just parts of a much larger "cluster" nut that grows readily in South American climates. The trees grow up to 150 feet tall and the nuts weigh three to four pounds each, crashing to the ground when ripe. Definitely a hard hat area. Once you've broken your hands getting the shell cracked, you'll find a whitish, oily nut which is worshipped by some and despised by others. Many a bag of mixed nuts has been reduced to a bag of Brazil nuts carefully avoided by seemingly inattentive munchers, while others rummage past the filberts and cashews to get at the Brazils.

Taste preferences aside, Brazils have their ups and downs. They are a good source of protein and particularly the sulfur-containing amino acids so often found in small amounts in vegetable proteins, but they contain quite a bit of saturated fat—third ranked in this category, after peanuts and coconuts.

Because of their generally high oil content, Brazils tend to get rancid more quickly than other nuts and should be checked over carefully before you buy. The nuts should be white or off-white and leave no bitter aftertaste in the back of the throat. Deep yellow nuts displayed on unrefrigerated shelves should be considered questionable at best.

Cashews

Although cashew nuts could be grown readily in several parts of the U.S., they are not, and all cashews sold here have been imported primarily from China, Africa, India, and South America.

Strictly speaking, there is no such thing as a "raw" cashew available commercially, since all cashews must be subjected to heat in order to get them out of their shells and to destroy a rather powerful toxin contained between the shell and the nut. This toxin can cause severe skin burning and, in sufficient doses, even poisoning. It is a little known fact that the cashew tree is related botanically to several other rash-producing species such as poison oak and poison sumac, and to a delicious tropical fruit, the mango, which is also known to cause acute skin rashes in certain sensitive individuals.

Despite this mandatory preroasting, you will still find cashews labeled "raw" and "roasted" for sale. The raw ones are "as raw as you can get," so to speak, having been subjected to no further heating after the initial processing. Additional roasting imparts that rich brown color and full taste enjoyed by so many.

Bad news for the purists: cashews are routinely treated with methyl bromide to halt or prevent insect infestation. There doesn't seem to be any practical way around this, since they are very popular with bugs and have to be stored and shipped for long periods of time. If you're concerned about keeping any and all chemicals out of your food, better strike cashews from your list.

Chestnuts

Chestnuts have never been exceptionally popular in the U.S., compared to almonds and cashews, but are recently experiencing a sort of revival due to popular interest in the low fat diet. Chestnuts are radically different from all other nuts with respect to their nutritional makeup. They are high in carbohydrate, low in fat, and low in calories.

Chestnuts may be eaten raw, but due to their high starch content taste better cooked. They may be boiled, steamed, baked, or, if you insist, roasted on an open fire.

Coconut

Probably no nut has found more uses in this world than the coconut. Besides all the nonedible uses such as in soaps and cosmetics, it finds its way into a huge variety of prepared and processed foods, usually in the form of coconut oil. This is unfortunate since coconut is not a very desirable food from a nutritional standpoint. Of all natural foods, it has the highest level of fat, practically all of which is saturated. It is 92 percent fat, far higher than even meat, eggs, or cheese, and contains relatively small amounts of vitamins and minerals.

Filberts

Known in some parts of the country as *Hazel nuts*, filberts are a fairly middle-of-the-road sort of nut, not especially high or low in calories, protein, and fats. Although they have a rich, full taste even raw, they have never approached the supermarket stardom of almonds, walnuts, and cashews. Most often they are just another participant in a nut mix, eaten along with the rest.

Macadamia Nuts

If price is an indicator, the macadamia is the ultimate gourmet nut. A perfectly round, small nut with an incredibly hard shell, it is grown mainly in the tropics or subtropics and most people never hear of them until they visit Hawaii. Best to forget them except as a delicacy. Besides being expensive, they are 93 percent fat, although most of that is monounsaturated.

Unless you are willing to shell them yourself, your chances of getting a fresh nut which has not begun its decline into rancidity are slim at best, and shelling a macadamia is one of the world's great physical challenges. Those of you who love a challenge will need a pair of pliers to hold the nut firmly in place, a hard surface to place it on, a hammer to smack it with, and good aim. The hard surface, incidently, should be concrete or steel, not your dining room table, unless you want it to look like the surface of the moon.

Macadamias are eaten raw or cooked, usually boiled in coconut oil, adding additional fat. They are generally used in treats such as cakes and ice cream. Despite all the nutritional misgivings, I confess to you that eating macadamia nut pie approaches a religious experience.

Peanuts

Since peanuts are actually peas and not nuts, they are discussed fully in Chapter 7.

Pecans

Also 93 percent fat, and also delicious, the pecan is the gourmet nut of the South. Prices generally run high on pecans, due often to their susceptibility to destruction by untimely frosts, not uncommon in areas like Georgia, Texas, and South Carolina, where pecans are grown.

Pecans may be purchased in the shell or out. As grown, pecan shells are a dull unimpressive brown. The ones you buy commercially have been polished and dyed to increase their attractiveness to some people.

Pecans are usually eaten raw as a snack or used in baked goods, including the famous pecan pie, possibly the world's highest calorie dessert.

Pine Nuts

Used more in European and Middle Eastern cookery, pine nuts, or *pignolias*, are exceptionally high in protein (22 percent) and moderate in fat (77 percent), for nuts that is. They grow inside the pine cones of certain species and are extracted by heating the cones moderately. They are available shelled and unshelled and are generally expensive enough to be considered a delicacy. They may be eaten raw or cooked in a variety of ethnic dishes.

Pistachio Nuts

Everyone knows what pistachio nuts look like, right? Bright red little guys that stain your fingers and lips, right? Wrong. Sorry to bring down another institution, but pistachios are light brown, not red. The red is dye, and it is used to cover up the mottled appearance pistachios get when they lay around on the ground too long. Dyeing gives them a nice uniform red color, so you can't tell the old ones from the fresh ones. Clever. A good natural food store should offer pistachios in the natural color, probably roasted and salted, roasted and unsalted, or raw and unsalted—take your pick.

One of Nature's little niceties is how when the pistachio ripens to maturity, the shell splits open at one end just enough for you to fit your thumbnail into it and pop it open. What Nature wasn't nice about is not allowing them to grow everywhere. Pistachio trees are confined to narrowly defined climatic regions, mainly in the Middle East—and like most things from the Middle East these days, the nuts are quite expensive. California is beginning to produce native pistachios, but so far afficionados feel they don't quite hold up to the Turkish and Iranian varieties.

Nutritionally, pistachios are about average in protein (12 percent of calories) and somewhat high in fat (81 percent of calories), but watch out mostly for the salt if you're eating the salted variety. You can take in an awful lot of sodium in a small bag of pistachios.

Walnuts

For baking, the walnut is second to none in popularity. Its full, meaty taste and chewy texture make it a natural for all kinds of cakes, pies, and cookies, and anyone who hasn't sampled maple walnut ice cream should be investigated. Whole unshelled walnuts are generally available all year, even in supermarkets. The shells have usually been bleached to prevent mold growth and produce uniform appearance, but this may be a harmless procedure unless you plan on eating the shells. Shelled walnuts are found in several forms: well-formed unbroken halves, halves and pieces, and diced. As always, the least fragmented form is best for freshness and stability.

Most of the walnuts we buy in America are California grown and are the English variety. Black walnuts are spoken of with hushed reverence in nutritional circles due to their somewhat higher protein content, but they are not widely available.

Nutritionally, walnuts are high in fat (81 percent), and low in protein (9 percent), although almost all the fat is unsaturated. Walnuts are also a good source of vitamin E.

Selection and Storage

Rancidity rules when you're dealing with high oil content foods, and selection and subsequent storage becomes, therefore, a critical issue. If you are buying shelled nuts, choose carefully. Look for signs of rancidity, like yellowing. If you're shopping in a bulk store, buy a small amount and taste them. If they remind you of bacon or burn the back of your throat, don't buy any more from that batch, and do the store owner a favor and let him know. This doesn't mean you have to boycott the store forever because all their stuff is rancid. The owner may well have gotten a bad case of nuts from his supplier and was unaware of it. Most owners don't go around testing all their products each time a new batch is opened—most of them are sick of looking at the stuff. If you ask (and *please* ask!), the owner or manager will probably let you taste a nut or two to check for their freshness. It's his right to refuse you, and he may have to if he's plagued by munchers, but it won't hurt to try.

Your best defense against rancidity is to buy nuts in as whole a form as possible, unshelled if you can spare the time, but at least unbroken, and to buy them from a place that sells a lot of them. A fast turnover is always the best assurance of freshness. I have seen small vitamin type stores with a dozen or so bags of almonds or cashews neatly lined up inside a display refrigerator, giving the impression of crisp, right-off-the-tree freshness. Three months later, the same bags are still sitting there, while the bulk store up the street that dumps almonds into an unrefrigerated bin has sold 2000 pounds in the same period. Which ones do you want?

Once you have purchased what you consider to be fresh-as-possible nuts, by all means don't take them home and throw them in the cupboard, or display them neatly in some nifty, designer glass jar with a cork top. Looks great on your kitchen counter, but you'll soon have spoiled nuts. Keep them in the refrigerator, they are perishables, just like butter and cheese and fruits and vegetables.

A far more serious problem than rancidity is mold. Mold on nuts, as on certain grains and peanuts, can produce a substance known as *aflatoxin,* a powerful carcinogen and not to be messed with. It results not so much from age, but from the careless exposure of nuts to moisture. Often you can see this mold merely by visual inspection, but problems arise when the nut has been coated with something or otherwise disguised, as in various candies, ice creams, cakes, and cookies. This does not mean everything with nuts in it is going to give you cancer; it is simply a call to be careful about prepared foods. It's always nicer to know what you are eating. Since aflatoxin produces liver cancer, and liver cancer is not that common in the U.S., the chances are that aflatoxin is not a problem of great proportions.

Seeds

Like nuts, seeds are considerably high in fat, mostly unsaturated, with protein values in the moderate range (13 to 20 percent of calories), but often are far better suppliers of important vitamins and minerals. Pumpkin seeds, for example, are quite high in iron and zinc, and sunflower seeds are high in potassium and B vitamins.

Considering the roughly equal amounts of fat and protein in nuts and seeds, the higher vitamin-mineral content of seeds, and the far lower cost (except for pumpkin), seeds stack up as the wiser choice of the two. A pound of sunflower seeds costs about one-third as much as the same amount of almonds and provide considerably more basic nutrition. However, you may like the taste of almonds better than sunflower seeds, in which case all of the above becomes irrelevant. Just thought you'd like to know.

Although several oilseeds could be used as human food, only three have achieved any measure of popularity.

Pumpkin Seeds

By far the most expensive, but probably the tastiest, of seeds, are the colorful green pumpkin seeds, or *pepitas* as they are sometimes called. They may be eaten raw or roasted and generally are found already shelled, though you can sometimes get them in the shell and spend all day getting them out.

Besides tasting good and being quite nutritious, pumpkin seeds are reputed to have the power of expelling worms in humans and animals. However, the process involves a total fast except for the seeds and some garlic. Not much fun, but then neither are worms.

Sesame Seeds

Sesame seeds are sold with or without hulls. The hulls, however, appear to contain quite a bit of a substance called calcium oxalate, which can have serious health effects, particularly with regard to the formation of kidney stones. Many foods contain oxalates, including rhubarb, spinach, and chard, but the quantities normally ingested are not considered harmful to the average person. The use of more than an ounce or two of unhulled sesame seeds on a daily basis might be excessive, however, and it is probably wisest to use the hulled variety.

An old mystery has recently been solved for me. For years I wondered how they managed to get those tiny hulls off sesame seeds. Being a child of the Industrial Age, I always operate on the assumption there are machines that can do anything, but how could they do it so inexpensively? Recently it came to my attention that these seeds are not hulled by machines at all but rather by chemical solvents. In other words, the hulls are *dissolved* in chemicals. Terrific. The chemical used is generally lye, and it appears to have a denaturing effect on the protein quality of the seed in addition to destroying various nutrients. Now a product called Protein-Aide has appeared on the market, and claims to be sesame seeds completely mechanically hulled, without chemicals. As you might expect they cost about double the price of regular sesame seeds.

Sunflower Seeds

These are generally the least expensive of the popular edible seeds. Like all seeds they are relatively high in fat, mostly unsaturated, moderate in protein, and contain some significant amounts of vitamins and minerals. Sunflower seeds are eaten raw or roasted, hulled or unhulled (they are mechanically hulled). The unhulled seeds make great sprouts (see Chapter 13), and the hulled seeds are easily digested and assimilated.

Selection and Storage

Everything that applies to nuts applies to seeds as well. Seeds can easily get rancid and should be inspected carefully. Pumpkin and sesame give off a definite "stale" odor when spoiled and sunflower turn yellow. If rancidity concerns you, as it should, you might want to take a few minutes, spread out your sunflower seeds and pick out any yellow ones. There will always be some. I've honestly never seen a sack of sunflower seeds that did not have some that had turned yellow.

Dried Fruit

Dried fruits are the "confection" of those who have given up or are struggling to give up sugar. They make great snacks for adults and kids, satisfy the sweet tooth, and provide that same "lift" of quick energy people try to get from candy bars and sodas.

The problem with dried fruits is that they are so concentrated a source of sugars and calories. If you ate a pound of dried apricots, you would have eaten the equivalent of six pounds of fresh apricots, and that equals about 1200 calories, most of which is fruit sugars. Now, it would be difficult for most of us to eat six pounds of fresh apricots, but a pound of dried ones is not that hard at all. And unless you're an athlete in training, that's probably a lot more extra calories and carbohydrates than you will be able to burn up in a day. Other fruits have higher or lower fresh to dried ratios (apples are 10 to 1; prunes 3 to 1).

For the average person without blood sugar problems, like diabetes or hypoglycemia, dried fruit in moderation is perfectly fine, and certainly preferable to the usual methods of placating the universal sweet tooth. The concept of moderation is critical here, as it is with all concentrated food.

Fruits are dried in a variety of ways. The simplest, most natural way is sun drying. This process doesn't lend itself well to large scale production, however, so you won't often find sun dried fruit available. Most of the fruit you will find has been dried in commercial dehydrators, where temperature and humidity are carefully controlled, the result being a more uniform and somewhat less nutritious product. Fruit is held at about 125° F for 24 hours or until the desired dry weight is achieved. Drying partially destroys vitamin A (carotene) and vitamin C, although using sulfur dioxide can offset some of these losses.

Which leads us to the subject of "sulfured" fruits. Many stores will deal only in unsulfured fruits, while others will offer a choice to the consumer. Sulfites of many types may be used as preservatives for dried fruits, but sulfur dioxide gas is the favorite. Introduced during the dehydration process, it helps the fruits retain their natural color, produces a softer, more palatable texture, and prevents some of the nutrient losses.

As far as sulfur dioxide residues go, they are presumed to be metabolized in the body and excreted harmlessly in the urine. After exhaustive testing, the Food and Drug Administration reports no negative effects from the intake of sulfites at certain levels. However, there is some question about their safety when large amounts of foods containing these preservatives are eaten, and it is best to minimize their use.

For some, there is no such thing as a safe or acceptable chemical, and they will have nothing to do with sulfured fruits. They prefer instead the leather-like, unsulfured fruits, which either need to be chewed much longer or even soaked overnight in water. Others couldn't care less about sulfur dioxide and like the soft, colorful, sulfured fruits far better.

The dried fruits you are likely to encounter include:

apples	mangos
apricots	nectarines
bananas	papaya
cherries	peaches

currants   pears
dates   pineapple
figs   prunes
           raisins

A few of these need special comments:

Dates

Of the dozens of available varieties, the most common are deglet noor, kadrawi, bread, halawi, zahidi, and the absolute queen of the date, medjool. Medjools grow quite large and can easily contain 50 calories each. Dates are usually dehydrated, but it is possible to find "hydrated" dates, i.e., not dried.

Figs

Again, there are many varieties, but you will most often encounter black mission figs or calmyrna figs ("white" figs). Each has a distinctly different taste and 1200 calories per pound.

Papaya

Except in Hawaii, it is hard to find papaya that hasn't been dipped in sugar or honey. This may not be stated on the label.

Pineapple

Most dried pineapple is soaked in sugar water and ends up about 80 percent sugar (sucrose). Even that labeled "honey dipped" is most likely sugared. Lately, however, some pineapple has been appearing on the market labeled "unsweetened." This means no sugar has been used but rather it is soaked in its own concentrate to increase sweetness. I have tasted real dried pineapple, completely untreated, and it is quite sour.

Raisins

The three most merchandised varieties are Thompson, Sultana, and Monukka. Thompson seedless are most common and are available organically grown, commercially grown (treated with potassium sorbate), and bleached until a golden yellow (called "golden raisins").

Monukkas are the best. A large, plump raisin with some tiny edible seeds inside, they have a most unique taste and have to be tried to be fully appreciated. They are more expensive, but worth it.

Sultanas are a reddish brown raisin rarely seen in the U.S.

Selection and Storage

Dried fruits are naturally preserved by the high concentrations of sugars within them, and although mold can form on them particularly if allowed to get moist, most dried fruits will keep fine out of refrigeration for several months. Dates are an exception, especially the nondehydrated types, and will ferment rather quickly in hot weather. The fermentation is harmless if you don't mind the wine-like taste and smell.

Lots of insects like dried fruits, especially raisins, so protecting them in a bug-proof container is not a bad idea, particularly if you live where cockroaches are prevalent.

Personally, I like to store any dried fruit which appears moist at all in the refrigerator rather than risk mold.

Fruits are generally harvested and dried at one time of the year and a steady supply is fed to the market throughout the year or as long as the stockpile lasts. If there were weather problems during the growing season, supplies of certain fruits may be short and they may not be around for the whole year. Needless to say, prices will fluctuate with availability. We have seen raisin prices double one year and halve the next, a function of farmer's problems with rain, frost, and storms.

Fruits dried in September may undergo certain natural changes over subsequent months. One of these is "sugaring," where tiny white crystals appear on the skin. People often think this is a mold growth of some kind, but it is actually just the solidifying and crystallization of the natural sugars in the fruit collecting on the surface. There is nothing wrong with these fruits.

One nice way to store dried fruits, especially the unsulfured kind, is in bottles of water in your refrigerator. Apricots, peaches, figs, and prunes in particular taste much better when soaked, and the liquid makes a great drink. Many feel they are far better for you this way since the added liquid makes them less dehydrating for the digestive system.

Nut, Seed, and Fruit Mixes

By far the most popular section of any natural food store is the bins or bags full of multicolored "trail mixes," "camp mixes," "energy mixes," or whatever other names you may have for them. They are basically some combination of nuts, seeds, and dried fruits thrown together and tossed like a salad. These mixes are often a person's first introduction to natural foods, and are great alternatives to junk food snacks.

Remember, though, that these are high energy foods. They have names like trail mix and camp mix because they are lightweight yet concentrated foods that you can nibble along the hiking trail and provide yourself with a steady stream of energy. But energy is just a polite way of saying calories. High energy means high calories, and if your idea of a hike is walking from the kitchen to the TV, trail mix is going to catch up with your waistline real fast. A pound of one of these mixes will run well over 2000 calories, and a pound isn't hard to put down. On the other hand, if you're determined to munch anyway, and carrot sticks and celery don't quite make it, trail mixes are a far better bet than most commercial treats.

Incidentally, for those who wish to gain weight for whatever reason, trail mixes are the way to go. They are nutritious, reasonably balanced, and a concentrated source of calories. Certainly better than milkshakes and protein powder.

Nut and Seed Butters

Although peanuts have long had the market cornered, any nut or seed may be ground into a butter. Granted, you don't get much call for walnut butter or filbert butter, but it is possible. For the most part we see almond butter, cashew butter, sesame seed butter, and of course, peanut butter. All of these are available in raw or roasted form already packed in neat little jars, but you can make your own at home using a food processor, certain kinds of juicers, a hand-cranked food mill, or even a blender. If you're using roasted nuts, just grind until you get the consistency you want. If you're interested in making a *raw* nut butter, you'll probably have to add some oil, since grinding raw nuts usually results in more of a powder than a butter. Whatever you make or buy should be refrigerated immediately after grinding or opening for the first time, since the finely ground particles are especially susceptible to rancidity.

Butters made from seeds are not nearly as popular as those from nuts, but one gaining a lot of ground these days is *tahini*, a butter made from sesame seeds and used in many Middle Eastern recipes, especially one called hummous, a dip and sandwich spread made from tahini and garbanzo beans.

Many natural food stores have grinders whereby customers may make their own peanut or other butters, in addition to stocking butters in jars. Grinding your own, whether it be at home or in the store, is always the best bet, since you can at least be sure it hasn't been sitting around in some bottling plant for days waiting to be packaged.

So what's so special about natural peanut butter? Well, for one thing it's made from 100 percent peanuts and that's all. Supermarket brands are often cut with hydrogenated fat and have added sugar and salt. And if you're grinding your own you can at least get a look at the peanuts going into it. Who knows what's going on at the peanut butter factory?

Fruit Butters and Preserves

It is un-American to talk about peanut butter without mentioning jelly. Natural food stores usually offer a good variety of jams, preserves, and fruit butters. Most are made with honey as a sweetener, although some are unsweetened, except for the natural sweetness of the fruit. These are pleasure foods, and no great nutritional claims should be made for them or expected from them.

Recipes

Nut and Seed Loaf

2 cups mixture of 2 or more of the following: almonds, cashews, walnuts, pecans, sunflower seeds, sesame seeds
1 large onion, chopped
2 egg whites
1 cup bulgur

1 cup cooked brown rice
2 Tbsp. salt-reduced tamari
½ tsp. garlic powder
1 tsp. dill weed
1 tsp. caraway seeds
Season to taste.

Blend nuts and seeds with tamari, egg whites, and just enough water to let blender work. Put in large bowl. Add remaining ingredients and mix thoroughly. Spoon and press into oiled loaf pan. Bake in 350° oven for 45 minutes. Serves 6–8.

Vegie-Nut Stir Fry

zucchini	mushrooms	raw almonds, cashews, walnuts
broccoli	carrots	soy or sesame oil
onions	peas	garlic
bell pepper	tomatoes	tamari to taste

Cut into chunks 8 cups of any combination of the above vegetables. Add garlic and 1 cup raw almonds, cashews and walnuts. Toss and stir fry in a small amount of soy or sesame oil and tamari. Serves 4.

Gado Gado (Indonesian Salad)

½ steamed cabbage
2 boiled potatoes, sliced
1 raw cucumber, sliced
1 cup steamed bean sprouts
3 stalks celery, sliced
1 cup tofu chunks

Sauce
½ cup peanut butter
¼ cup water
2 cloves garlic, chopped
1 tsp. ginger, ground
1 tsp. tamari

Mix sauce ingredients together and cook over low flame in open saucepan for 3–4 minutes, keeping extra water close by to add if sauce starts to thicken too quickly. Arrange vegetables and tofu creatively and spread hot sauce over top. Serves 2–3.

Peanut, Tofu, and Sesame Soup[9]

¾ cup raw peanuts, cooked
6 oz tofu, cut in ½" cubes
¼ cup chopped celery
¾ cup chopped onions
½–1 cup chopped mushrooms
4 cups stock, from cooking peanuts
2 cups canned tomatoes
1 cup sesame seeds, ground and roasted
soy or sesame oil
1 Tbsp. miso
¼ tsp. dried chili peppers
1 bay leaf

Spread the cooked peanuts on a large cutting board and chop them coarsely. Set aside. Using a small amount of oil, sauté the tofu cubes with the celery, onions, and mushrooms. The tofu should brown lightly and the onions should be golden. Combine the sautéed vegetables and tofu with the chopped peanuts in a pot. Stir in the peanut stock, tomatoes, and roasted sesame seeds. Add seasonings, simmer 20–25 minutes. Add miso and dissolve after cooking is over. Makes about 2 quarts.

Sun Dip[4]

¾ cup lemon juice
1 Tbsp. tamari
1 Tbsp. honey
1 Tbsp. paprika

1 tsp. basil
½ chopped red onion
2 cloves garlic, crushed
1½ cups sunflower seeds

Mix all ingredients together until well blended. Use as dip for raw vegetables or crackers.

Q. *I can handle this thing at home OK, but we like to go out to restaurants occasionally. What do we do then?*

A. If you're near a major city, there is probably a natural food restaurant available. If not, look for a restaurant with a good salad bar. They seem to be everywhere these days. Have a big salad and a couple of baked potatoes. Cheat a little—have some sour cream and chives—you'll never miss the prime ribs.

Ethnic restaurants are another possibility. Chinese, Indian, and Middle Eastern menus usually have vegetarian entrees not loaded down with cheese, butter, and eggs. They will more than likely be made with white rice, but this is less important than the fat content. At an Italian restaurant you can order pasta with a marinara (meatless) sauce and a salad, and if you're lucky enough, you might find a Mexican restaurant that does not use pork fat in their beans.

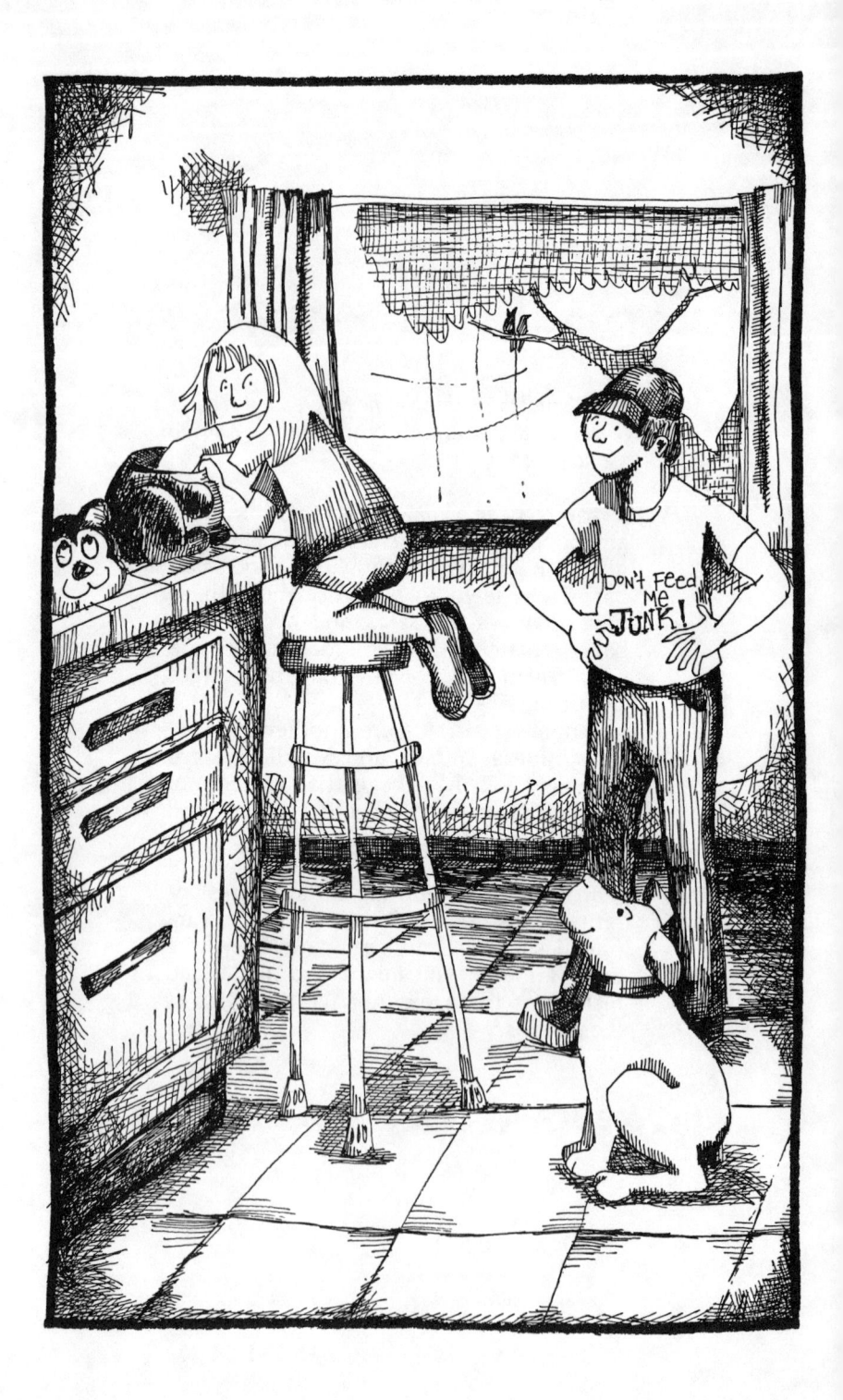

CHAPTER 12
Snacks

Americans and other Western peoples are the champs when it comes to snacking—there's no getting around that fact. And the natural food industry has not tried to get around it, they've aimed straight for it. So-called natural snacks make up an important percentage of the sales in any natural food store, and without them the industry would probably not exist.

As long as we've faced up to the fact that we may be occasional munchers, we can at least endeavor to munch healthier snacks. The idea behind the natural snack is to substitute and eliminate. Substitute the "bad" with the "good," or at least with the "less bad." Whole wheat flour for white flour, natural sweeteners for refined sugar, carob for chocolate, natural colors and flavors for artificial. Eliminate the preservatives, stabilizers, emulsifiers, and hydrogenated fats. All this is designed to produce a palatable snack, which although often no lower in calories, sugars, and fats, leaves the impression one is getting a far better product for his money, and for the most part he is.

Natural snacks serve a number of important functions for both the store owner and the consumer. We'd all probably be better off eating simple foods. But it would be extremely difficult for a store to survive today's high rents, insurance rates, utilities, and minimum wage laws selling rice and beans. Snacks pay the rent, plain and simple. Without them the bulk stores would cease to exist, and this would be a loss for everyone. What I am saying to the purist customer I suppose is: Don't be hard on your store for selling carob-coated malt balls and candy bars; without them there would be no natural food stores and you'd be forced back to the supermarkets. What I am saying to the store owner is: Admit to yourself that these are not the best foods for your customers, and although you have to sell them don't make them out to be any better than they actually are.

Snacks are the perfect "transition" food, and often represent the first contact a person has with natural foods. Once a newcomer has tried and enjoyed a "natural snack," he begins to discard the stereotype that anything that's good for you has to taste bad. "Hey . . . (with great surprise) . . . this stuff is pretty good!" It's almost as if he expects everything in a health food store to taste like yeast and cod liver oil.

Anyhow, the theory is that someone who tries a snack and likes it might be persuaded to try other natural foods and before you know it he's buying whole wheat bread, fresh peanut butter, unfiltered juices, alfalfa sprouts, and, Heaven forbid, even green spaghetti.

I would venture to say that very few natural food purists did not follow a similar line of development in their transition from junk food to real food.

Snacks are "good news—bad news" foods, and they fall roughly into two distinct categories, based upon whether their bad news is sweet or salty. Let's face it, a snack is a snack because it stimulates and satisfies, at least temporarily, a craving. One doesn't snack on brown rice—one sits down and eats brown rice for dinner, lunch, or even breakfast, but you don't watch a ball game or a drive-in movie happily popping kernels of brown rice into your mouth.

The cravings for which satisfaction is most often sought are for something sweet or something salty. Neither of these cravings is good and every effort should be made to control them. But if you have them, and if you're going to give way to them occasionally, it might as well be with the least harmful food you can find.

Sweet Snacks

The main good news about sweet natural food snacks is the lack of chemical additives, although this is not always the case and careful label reading is advised. In some cases lower calories and fat is also a good news factor. The bad news is sugar. Sweets don't get sweet on their own, and usually a sweetening agent is added. Sweeteners run the gamut: white sugar, brown sugar, raw sugar, malt syrup, fructose, maple syrup, honey, molasses, date sugar, and so forth. As we already know from Chapter 10, the differences between these are inconsequential. Sugar is sugar. People often naively believe that nothing in a natural food store contains sugar. I have seen stores idealistically try to exclude all sugar products from their shelves, but they didn't stay open very long. If you want to avoid refined sugars totally you'd better stick with fruit as your snack.

Carob

Of all the sweet snacks available, *carob* is unquestionably the king. Carob is produced from the carob bean and makes an excellent substitute for chocolate, having a very similar taste but considerably more nutrition. A hundred grams (about 3½ ounces) of carob powder provides 4.5 grams of protein, only 1.5 grams of fat, and 180 calories. The same amount of plain chocolate yields 4.1 grams of protein, 30.6 grams of fat, and 534 calories. In addition, carob contains a large amount of fiber and about seven times the calcium of chocolate. The fat in chocolate is predominately saturated, more so than that in beef and second only to coconut. All this makes carob an attractive alternative to chocolate for those who have acquired the habit and want to at least soften the impact a bit.

Since carob has grown in popularity it has been used to coat or flavor just about everything. Carob-coated peanuts, almonds, cashews, filberts, pecans, raisins, dates, pineapple, sunflower seeds, soybeans, malt balls, etc. Carob chips are substituted for chocolate chips in cookies, carob milk for chocolate milk—carob syrup, carob ice cream, carob yogurt, carob everything.

Now, it would be nice if a carob-coated peanut, for example, were just a peanut with nice, natural carob wrapped around it, but this is not the case. Things have to be added to the carob to make it behave the way we want it to. Carob coating usually contains whey (a part of milk), lecithin, hydrogenated oil, and some kind of sweetener, usually sugar, but sometimes fructose, date sugar, malt, or honey. I have seen a line of carob products using no sweeteners, depending upon the natural sweetness of carob and perhaps milk sugar.

Yogurt Coating

The same foods that have been coated with carob for years are now being coated with "yogurt"—actually not yogurt but a combination of ingredients including yogurt, sugar, whey, lecithin, and often artificial color or flavor.

Banana Chips

Manufactured primarily in the Philippines, banana chips have become an extremely popular snack. Again, there is more than meets the eye here, for what might be assumed to be merely slices of cooked and dried bananas usually contains honey and/or raw sugar, vegetable oil of unspecified variety, and often artificial flavor. Watch your labels.

Candy Bars

Hundreds and hundreds of "natural" candy bars are offered today, from the traditional Tiger's Milk protein bars to complicated conglomerations of ingredients touted to get you up and down Mt. Everest with energy to spare. It would be pointless to discuss the ingredients of each of these, but a few things should be pointed out.

First, don't be taken in by all this "natural" and "organic" talk on the label—read the ingredients. If you're trying to cut back on sugars, watch for the disguises: sucrose, dextrose, corn syrup, fructose 90, malt syrup, invert sugar, glucose. If fats are your special concern, look out for "partially hydrogenated palm kernel oil" or "partially hydrogenated cottonseed and palm oil," and of course good old coconut oil. And don't be shocked if you see an artificial color or flavor thrown into your "natural, organic" candy bar. Lots of people out there are trying to make money on this movement, and their levels of integrity range from high to zero.

Second, a candy bar is a candy bar, and it is going to be packed with calories regardless of how organic it is. Don't walk around munching on bars all day and wonder how you got fat eating health food.

Now that I've made enemies of every candy manufacturer in the country, let me make friends with a few. If you look around carefully, you can find "candy bars" made with totally natural ingredients and no added sugars or fats. These are made from nuts, seeds, and dried fruits, blended and pressed together into a bar or ball, and depend only upon their raisins or dates for sweetness. Switching to these would definitely be a step toward a better diet.

Salty Snacks

The good news here is no chemicals. The bad news is high salt and high oil content. Basically there is only one salty snack, the potato chip, and all others are derived from it in spirit. Take something starchy (potato, wheat, corn, soy), fry it in oil, and salt it up. So we have corn nuts, cheddar chips, sesame stix, wheat nuts, soynuts, and so forth. The ingredients vary from snack to snack but the basic structure remains: starch, oil, salt.

Generally these snacks are cooked in a better quality oil that is not hydrogenated. Often they list "wheat flour" as their primary ingredient. What does that mean? Whole wheat? I doubt it. Probably white flour.

It is possible to find snacks that have been neither oiled nor salted, like plain soynuts or toasted soybeans, but one wonders whether they can any longer qualify as snacks.

Storage

Carob goodies really don't require refrigeration, but they will melt in the sun or in hot places, and they will attract critters, so keep them well protected.

Remember, as always, where there's oil there's rancidity, so any products cooked in oil or otherwise oil treated should be eaten right away or refrigerated. Better yet, forgo them altogether.

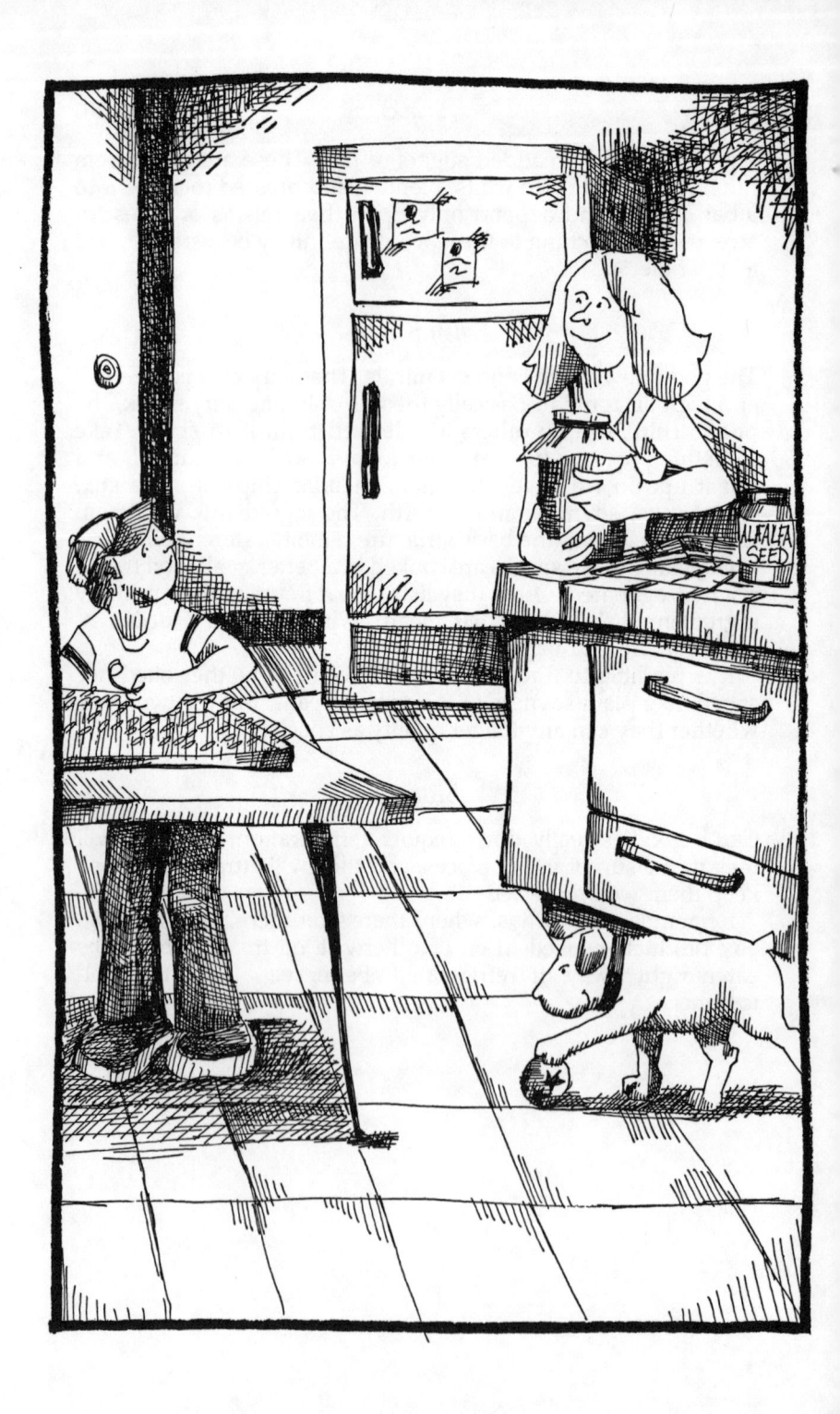

CHAPTER 13

Sprouts

Sprouts are one food I can give an unqualified endorsement. They are highly nutritious, economical, fun, and as close as you can get to a guaranteed organic food, and a "live" one at that.

For most people sprouts mean bean sprouts and Chinese restaurants, or maybe those funny little alfalfa things they put on sandwiches in health food restaurants. But as you will find, there are dozens of seeds which may be sprouted and eaten, each one having its own unique flavor and texture.

Nutrition

If you measure the nutritional value of a seed, sprout that seed, and measure the nutritional value of the sprout after a few days, you will find that the amounts of protein, vitamins, and minerals have vastly increased. This is a live and growing food, gathering nutrients from the air, sun, and water, undergoing a myriad of complicated biochemical changes, and producing a new organism. It is the plant world's version of pregnancy.

The final product of this process is a highly digestible and assimilable storehouse of nutrients. Sprouts have the nutrient value of greens rather than the seeds they emerged from. Soybean sprouts, for example, are more like broccoli than soybeans, although not quite as good in vitamins and minerals as broccoli. A sprout derived from a grain would be nutritionally similar to lettuce, and therefore would not replace grains in the diet. Sprouts are low calorie foods, great for the overweight, but don't expect to live on them exclusively. The important thing to know is that if you were ever stuck in a concentration camp and given grains, you could sprout them and produce a green food containing enough vitamin A and C to at least avoid major deficiency diseases like scurvy.

Yet, there is perhaps something more here. This "live food," raw in every sense of the word, also contains a host of enzymes essential to the life and growth of the plant. Do these enzymes have any health promoting effects on the human system? On this issue, opinions and philosophies predominate over facts. One side says flatly that all such enzymes are destroyed by the hydrochloric acid in the stomach, so their potential value to the human system, even if there is any, is irrelevant and academic.

The opposition believes, with religious fervor, that all living forms are related, and that the plant enzymes are critically important for maintaining vital health in the human species. All healthy diets throughout the world include large amounts of raw and living foods, they point out, and cooking destroys the essential integrity of our sustenance. The leading proponent of this point of view is the Hippocrates Institute, headquartered in Boston, Mass. The institute deals with cancer patients and others suffering from other degenerative diseases who have "given up," to some degree, on doctors and medical science in the search for salvation from their disease. Often these people have been told by their physicians that they are terminal and have only short periods of time to live, barring Divine intervention. The Hippocrates Institute intervenes and claims to save a good many patients, by first putting them on a 100 percent raw food diet, with no animal products. Food is organically grown and free from artificial chemical residues. Sprouts make up a large part of the diet, and these living foods are given credit for great healing. Although many varieties of sprouts are used, the star is undeniably *wheatgrass*, a grass-like sprout from wheat "berries" (wheat seeds) grown in trays containing an inch or two of high quality, composted soil, with even a few earthworms crawling about. After this grass is six or seven inches high, it is cut down and put through heavy duty juicers, producing wheatgrass juice, a thick chlorophyll green liquid that is drunk on a regular schedule throughout the day, or even "implanted." rectally.

Bizarre as it may seem, the institute claims to get good results from this type of therapy, although there are no genuine scientific studies supporting this view. One could, of course, argue that the increase in faith and will to live are powerful psychosomatic agents even capable of putting cancer into remission, and that herein lies the true value of such therapies. On the other hand, there is much science does not know about the mysteries of nature, and wheatgrass and live food may very well be something to believe in.

By the way, you may occasionally see wheatgrass juice for sale in tiny containers, at exorbitant prices. Don't bother. Chances are the enzymes and nutrients have long been lost through exposure to air and light, leaving little more than an expensive breath freshener. If you want to use wheatgrass, you'll have to grow it yourself, juice it, and drink it on the spot for maximum benefit.

Economics

Time was when a serious vegetarian could live on 25 cents a day. Not anymore, with the cost of green vegies getting higher and higher. Why not grow your own salad vegetables at home? Sprouts are the perfect solution: no land, no digging, no fertilizing, no frost damage, no insects, and no waiting. Your initial investment may be nil, or a few dollars at best. Sprouting is a way you can easily produce nutritious vegetables for as little as 5 to 10 cents a pound.

Fun

Sprouting and children are a perfect combination. It's easy enough for any child to handle, and he has a science lesson, economics lesson, an appreciation of nutritious food, and lunch, all at once.

How To Sprout

All you really need for sprouting are some seeds, water, and a means of drainage whereby you can keep the seeds moist but not drowning. This could be done on a piece of screen, in a colander or strainer, or even on several layers of paper towels; but everyone's favorite is the sprouting jar. Any old jar will do as long as it has a wide mouth and at least a quart capacity. The mayonnaise jar is traditional. Now all you need is some sort of screen to fit over the mouth so that water can be poured in and drained out leaving only moistened seeds or young sprouts in the jar. Natural food stores will sell you custom made plastic caps with screened openings tailored to fit the standard mayonnaise jar; just snap them on and you're ready to go. They'll even sell you the jar if you're not into mayonnaise. If a dollar or so for a sprouting lid offends your pioneer spirit, you can use a piece of cheesecloth and a rubberband. I find the screen to work best since cheesecloth and nylon tend to get moldy after a short while and have to be replaced.

Next, choose some seeds to sprout. I recommend alfalfa or mung beans for the first try since they seem to be the most problem free. Figure on about two tablespoons of seeds for a quart jar, put your seeds in the jar, add two or three inches of water and let them soak overnight.

In the morning, put your screen on the jar and dump out the water, add more water and rinse seeds thoroughly, dumping out the final water, leaving only dampened seeds with no puddles. Now shake the jar until the seeds spread out over one side, trying to avoid big clumps of wet seeds. The jar, laying on its side, can be placed on a counter or shelf and let be. It used to be thought that the seeds needed darkness to germinate properly, but this is no longer believed; in fact it has been determined that a better balance of nutrients is achieved when sprouts are grown in indirect sunlight. An area where good air circulation exists is also quite important to prevent molding. If you do a lot of sprouting you may want to build a shelf or two to hold lots of jars with different sprouts in different stages of growth.

Next, your developing sprouts need to be rinsed regularly. How often you do this depends on where you live. You may have to rinse three or four times a day in Phoenix, Ariz., but only once or twice a day in Miami, Fla. In other words, the more humidity in the air, the less you should water, since excessive moisture will promote mold.

In most areas of the country, where humidity is not extreme, two or three rinsings a day works well. Obviously you have to experiment a little to get the right balance. But rather than methodically follow a watering schedule, it's best to just look over your sprouts and decide if they need water. Basically you treat them like house plants. You want them to be moist but not wet, and certainly not dry. Just play with it a little and you'll soon be an expert.

After a few days your seeds will become sprouts and little yellow leaves will appear, and soon after the diffuse sunlight will start the photosynthetic processes which turn the yellow leaves green and add nutrients. After a day of this, your little friends are ready to eat. You may have gotten to know them on a first name basis by now and feel guilty about devouring them.

Not to worry, they like being eaten. They also like being kept in the refrigerator by the way, and not in an airtight container—they need to breathe.

Some people like to rinse away the hulls. This is not necessary, however, it may help prevent molding. This may be accomplished by switching your sprouting lid with a special one with larger holes which the hulls but not the sprouts will fall through; or just soak your sprouts in a bowl of water and the hulls will float away.

If the jar technique doesn't appeal to you, your local store will gladly show you all sorts of sprouting utensils, costing up to $10 or more, which are quite nice and make sprouting even easier.

Now that you're an expert on sprouting alfalfa and mung, you should try some of the other seeds until you develop a repertoire that is suited to your taste preferences. Here's a partial list of other seeds that may be sprouted in a jar and are usually available in natural food stores.

radish	hulled sunflower seeds
Chinese cabbage	unhulled sesame seeds
black mustard	all whole grains
fenugreek	all beans
red clover	

One question that often arises is how long to let sprouts grow before harvesting. For the most part, sprouts have reached their nutritional peak in three or four days and letting them grow any longer will not result in any significant gains. Not only that, but they tend to get tougher and chewier as they get longer. Grains especially should get only about ¼ inch of sprout before you eat them, since they get awfully tough and "grassy" tasting. Also, certain beans, like garbanzos and pintos, should only grow to a short length.

There are two other types of sprouts that you cannot do in a jar. The *muscillagenous* seeds, like chia, flax, and cress, form a mucous-like gel when soaked and will never sprout out of this mess, only spoil. They are best spread out on a plate or a wooden bowl and sprayed with water using a plant "mister." Another technique is to soak thoroughly in water a porous container, like a clay flower pot; soak the seeds for ½ hour or so, just to make them sticky enough to adhere to the sides of the pot; and stick the seeds along the outside surface of the pot. The water held in the clay will feed your sprouts as they grow. If it gets dry, just fill with water with your finger over the drainage hole, and it will soak itself again.

The final type of sprout requires a bit more work. Buckwheat and sunflower are both grown best on soil, the same way as wheatgrass. Seeds are soaked overnight and placed in trays containing an inch or two of soil, usually blended with peat moss or compost. The seeds are simply spread over the top soil, not tamped in, covered with newspaper or dark plastic for a couple of days until growth begins and then uncovered to flourish in diffuse and direct sunlight. The soil is soaked thoroughly before adding the seeds, and periodic watering is done only as needed, i.e., enough to keep the soil *moist*. Sprouts should be four or five inches high in a week or less and are ready to be harvested, rinsed, and refrigerated.

Sprouting buckwheat is what you want for this, with the black hull still on. It will produce what is often called "buckwheat lettuce," a four-leaf clover type plant that is delicious in salads or on sandwiches. Unhulled sunflower seeds will yield miniature sunflower plants with big green leaves, also excellent salad greens. Sunflower sprouts have a little sharp bite to them and this increases as the sprout grows, so you can decide on the basis of your own taste when to cut them. And if you are interested in growing wheatgrass, it is done in precisely the same way. Don't plan on putting it in your salad though. Wheatgrass is as tough as nylon and quite inedible, although you can chew on it to extract the juice and spit the fibers out.

After soil-sprouts have been harvested, the root-filled soil should be dumped into a composting barrel and churned up for later recycling. Continuous composting and recycling will produce an increasingly better soil and hence better crops. Your own little ecosystem right on the back porch.

Most sprouting books recommend old baker's trays for this type of work, but they don't seem all that easy to come by anymore. I prefer those plastic trays from plant nurseries that they use for starting plants. They're about 12" × 24" × 3" and cost less than $1 each.

Use of Sprouts

What do you do with them now that you've got them? The best thing is the simplest: just eat them raw, right out of the sprouting bottle. A variety of sprouts are great thrown into a salad or used on a sandwich. You can stir-fry them in wok-style dishes, or bake them into vegetarian meat loaves. Sprouted breads are becoming quite popular. These are made from wheat sprouts run through a grinder and baked along with traditional bread ingredients, or all by themselves in a simple unyeasted flatbread.

Sprouting Guide

Seed	Dry Measure	Yield	Soak Time	Growing Time*	Harvest Length
Alfalfa	2 Tbsp.	1 quart	4–6 hours	4–6 days	1–2 inches
Blackeyed Peas	1 cup	1 quart	8–12 hours	3–4 days	¼–¾ inch
Cabbage	¼ cup	1 quart	8–12 hours	4–6 days	¾–1½ inches
Corn	1 cup	1 quart	12–16 hours	3–8 days	½–1 inch
Garbanzos	¾ cup	1 quart	12–16 hours	3–5 days	½–1 inch
Lentils	¾ cup	1 quart	3–12 hours	3–4 days	¼–½ inch
Mung Beans	½ cup	1 quart	8–12 hours	3–5 days	½–2 inches
Radish	¼ cup	1 quart	8–12 hours	3–5 days	½–1½ inches
Soybeans	1 cup	1 quart	12–16 hours	3–5 days	½–1 inch
Sunflower	2 cups	1 quart	8–12 hours	2–3 days	½ inch
Wheat	1¼ cups	1 quart	8–12 hours	2–3 days	¼ inch

*Growing time will vary with temperature and water condition.

Recipes

Sprout Bread

Sprout wheat until sprouts are ¼ inch long. Run through a meat grinder or Champion juicer. Form into a mound about 8 inches in diameter and 2–3 inches high. Bake at 200°F until bread springs back when poked.

Alfalfa Dip

1 cup alfalfa sprouts
⅓ cup olive oil
½ cup lemon juice
2 Tbsp. chopped celery
2 Tbsp. chopped onion
2 Tbsp. ground sesame seeds
2 Tbsp. honey
½ tsp. tamari

Blend. Use as a dip for raw vegetables or crackers.

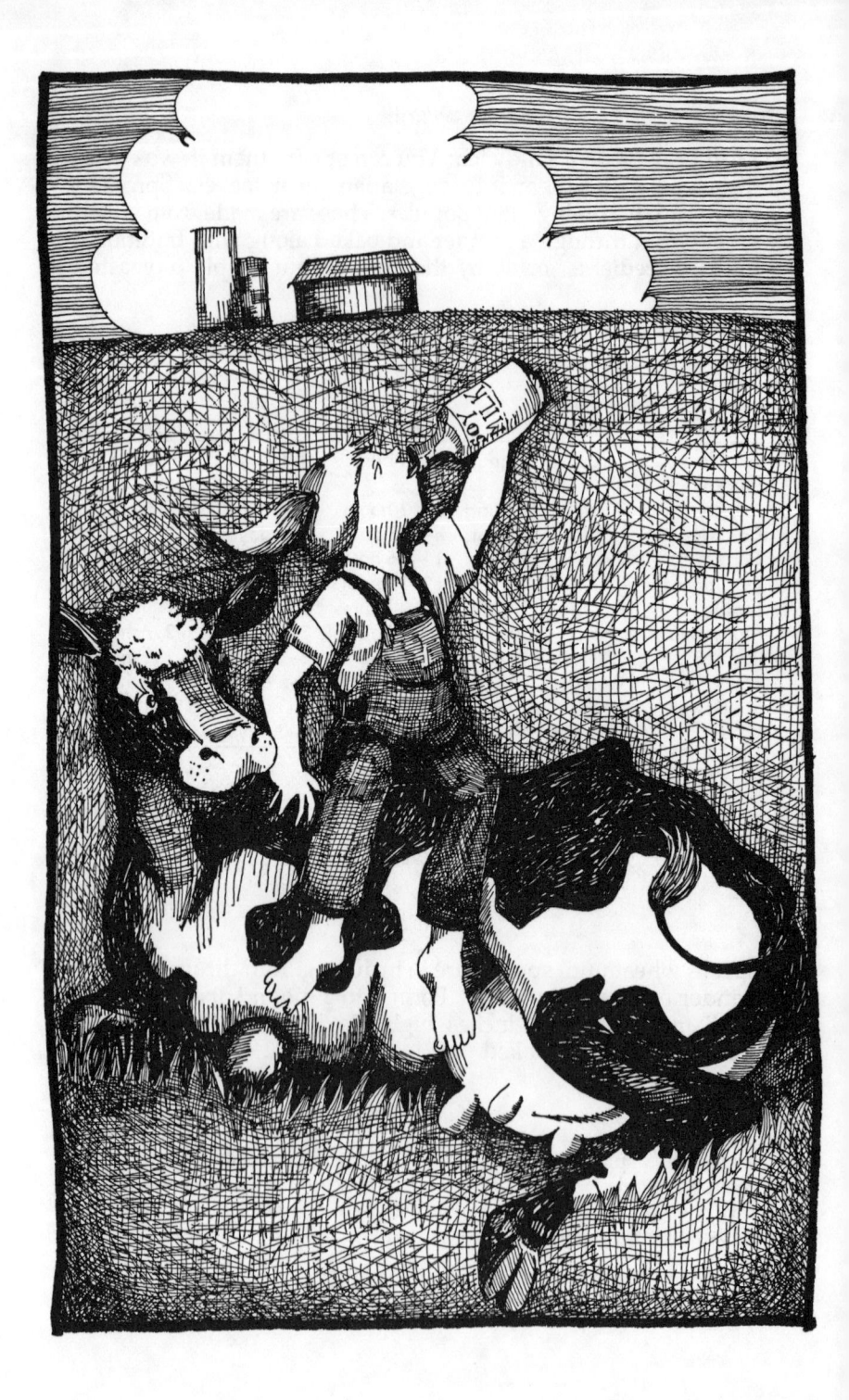

CHAPTER 14

Dairy Products, Eggs, and Substitutes

Natural food shops abound with dairy products of every conceivable type. The amount and scope of dairy a store carries is limited only by how much refrigeration they can afford. Some stores do not have the space nor the capital to put in cumbersome and expensive, glass door, reach-in coolers and freezers and may therefore have to keep their dairy line to the essential minimum and/or use secondhand "home kitchen" appliances. But there is definitely no shortage of companies manufacturing and distributing milk and egg products.

The first question you may legitimately ask is what is the difference between the dairy products you buy in a natural food store and those from the supermarket? After all milk still comes from cows and eggs from chickens, right? Right. But what kind of cows and chickens, and how the products are processed and adulterated on their way to your refrigerator is the central issue.

Probably the prime difference is additives. Commercial cheeses, yogurts, butters, and especially ice creams are routinely assaulted with emulsifiers, stabilizers, artificial colors, artificial flavors, and preservatives, while their natural food counterparts do not contain these relatively unnecessary and possibly harmful ingredients.

The sugar issue enters here of course. Commercial yogurts and ice creams contain plenty of it. The natural ones use honey, but we know what that's all about.

A third difference, in states where laws allow it, is the availability of *certified raw milk*. Raw milk has not been subjected to pasteurization, a process highly destructive of enzymes, vitamins and proteins, that also may bind up a significant amount of the calcium into insoluble, and therefore unuseable, compounds. Certified raw milk is produced in dairies where continuous government and medical inspection takes place and standards of cleanliness are extremely high—far higher I might add than those set for ordinary dairies, the assumption being, I suppose, that as long as you're going to pasteurize the product anyhow, why worry too much about how clean it is.

The arguments against raw milk are clear. Cows get diseases, or at least they get disease-producing organisms into their systems, and these can be transmitted to humans through the milk. Nasty stuff like salmonella and staphylococcus are seen to be lurking everywhere, and perhaps they are. And then there's tuberculosis. Peoples' worries about TB as well as brucellosis come up often during discussions of raw milk. Another concern is Q-fever virus, which was found not to be destroyed by the old pasteurization technique using a temperature of 142° F for 30 minutes. The new method involves higher heat (161° F) for only 15 seconds.[1] Raw milk dairies claim to have solved all these problems simply by keeping their herds healthy, and I have no reason to believe that is not true, since the government keeps a particularly vigilant watch over them. The big problem of the future is the leukemia virus which has recently been shown to be transmitted through raw milk,[2] but of course a healthy animal should not have leukemia either.

Raw milk continues to be produced and marketed in some places, although government pressures increase daily to force dairies to pasteurize or close down. For the moment, however, the choice still belongs to the consumer in these parts of the country.

Finally, the quality of the animal may be worth mentioning. Does a cow produce healthier milk if it is free to graze naturally, fed pesticide-free grain, and not cramped up in a milk factory pen, force-fed, and pumped full of steroids and antibiotics? Does a hen lay a better egg if fed pure grain and allowed to run around the henyard freely and consort with roosters rather than being kept five or six to a tiny cage on a continuous light cycle to beef up laying? Although comparative nutrient analyses show no difference, all the facts upon which to decide this issue are probably not in yet.

To my way of thinking, it makes a difference, possibly a big difference. Just as the quality of a newborn infant depends on

Dairy Products, Eggs, and Substitutes

the proper nutrition and emotional health of its mother, so I believe does the quality of an egg or milk depend on the relative health of its producer.

With all this in mind, let's now look at some of the dairy products available from natural food stores and how they compare to those sold in conventional markets.

Dairy Products

Milk

Supermarket milk usually contains added synthetic or natural vitamins A and D. These are tossed in on the assumption that most people have such lousy diets they are deficient in these vitamins. If you're eating yellow fruits and green vegetables, you need not worry about vitamin A, and if you get yourself out in the sun ten minutes a day during the summer, you'll get all the vitamin D you need for the year. These additional vitamins are probably not harmful, just unnecessary, and certainly do not result in a balanced food. Vegetarians may be interested in knowing that the vitamin D sometimes used is vitamin D3 from fish liver oil.

If a natural food store sells milk at all, it is probably raw milk, goat's milk, or some "novelty" milk, like carob flavored or acidophilus milk, rather than just ordinary pasteurized cow's milk.

Goat's milk is either pasteurized or raw. The raw version probably is not medically certified, and therefore its safety is solely a function of the care taken by the goat tender who supplies it. If goats are kept healthy and fed properly, and equipment is sterilized, the milk is safe to drink. Otherwise you may be taking a chance. In states where raw milk is illegal, raw goat milk is sometimes sold with a warning "not fit for human consumption," or "for pet food only." This protects the producer and the merchant. What the consumer does with it is his own business.

Lots of people drink goat's milk because they have allergies to cow's milk and feel they need some kind of milk in their diets, although we know this to be untrue. Others drink goat's milk because they consider it nutritionally superior. A cult has developed around goat's milk, and all sorts of special powers are attributed to it, none of which are supported by scientific evidence. Nutritional analyses show little if any difference between cow's and goat's milk, except perhaps that goat's milk contains more fat, which is certainly not an advantage.

Acidophilus milk has been cultured with *lactobacillus acidophilus*, a yeast-like micro-organism which "sours" the milk while breaking down some of the protein, making it more digestible. For this reason, it may be used by some people with mild milk allergies, since their problem is often difficulty digesting milk protein.

Cheese

You know that nice, bright orange cheddar cheese you see smiling out at you from the supermarket dairy coolers and fancy imported cheese shops? Ever wonder how it got so orange? After all, cheese is made from milk and I don't know of any cow that gives orange milk. I suppose it's from the aging process, right? Wrong. It's artificial coloring and you have been tricked again. Any cheese you purchase in a natural food store should be white or pale yellow and therefore uncolored.

Both pasteurized and raw milk cheese will no doubt be available. Raw milk cheese is not raw in the strict sense; some heat must be applied in the making of cheese, and therefore it may be sold in places where raw milk is banned. A good raw milk cheese, made by a reputable manufacturer should be heated no higher than 120° F. This temperature, combined with a federally imposed sixty day minimum aging period, serves to eliminate potentially dangerous bacteria yet is not so severe as to destroy essential nutrients.

Supermarkets sell several types of cheeses, the least objectionable of which are labeled "natural cheese." This may be dyed and contain a preservative or two, but will otherwise be unadulterated, although undoubtedly made from pasteurized milk. A second class of cheese is called "processed cheese." Processed cheeses are heated to stop the ripening process, making for more convenient shipping and long-term storage without spoilage. Emulsifiers and stabilizers are added, and generally coloring and flavoring. In all, up to thirteen chemicals may be added to "pasteurized processed cheese," better known to most of us as American Cheese. A third class of cheese is so adulterated it may no longer be called cheese. This is "cheese food." The same chemicals added to processed cheese are here, and some of the cheese itself has been removed and replaced with milk or cream and water.

Another new word you will come across in the natural food store cheese department is *"rennetless."* In order for milk to become cheese it must have a coagulant added to it. This is an enzyme which induces curdling of the milk protein and most of its fat. The curd is then separated from the whey (mostly water and milk sugar), and proceeds to ripen into cheese. The coagulant most commonly used is *rennet*, an enzyme from the stomach of a cow. Some people prefer not to eat the enzyme and will seek out rennetless cheese, which is made through microbiological action. I know of no valid health reason to avoid rennet, particularly if you're eating an animal product like cheese anyway. However, most objections to rennet are philosophical and based on the fact that the cow must be slaughtered to obtain the enzyme.

Commercial cottage cheese generally contains a number of additives, sometimes including an interesting one called *diacetyl*, which might be rightfully termed an "artificial odor," since it gives the aroma of butterfat, thus allowing the manufacturer to dilute the cottage cheese with water and cut costs. Sneaky. Makers of natural cottage cheese resort to no such deception, and the product is pure. Needless to say, you'll pay for the difference. Although most cottage cheeses will be made with rennet, some may use an acidophilus culture, such as is used in producing yogurt, which yields a slightly tarter taste.

Finally, a number of what we might call "special diet" cheeses may be available at your natural food store. These will be such items as low fat cheese, low sodium cheese, and goat's milk cheese. The term low fat cheese is a bit misleading. "Lower fat cheese" might be more appropriate, since although cheese made with part skim milk is indeed lower in fat than that made from whole milk, it is by no means a low fat food. Whereas full fat cheese is 65 percent fat (by calories), low fat or part skim cheese is 53 percent fat, so you are still dealing with a fatty food. All this means is that if you are allotting yourself a certain number of grams of fat per day, you can allow a little more of the low fat cheese.

Low sodium cheese, on the other hand, is exactly what it says. At 12 mg of sodium per ounce, a low sodium cheddar cheese represents a significant reduction in salt intake when compared to ordinary cheddar cheese, at 176 mg per ounce—a fourteen-fold difference, and a definite plus for those on sodium-restricted diets.

Goat's milk cheese is eaten by the same people who drink goat's milk, and no doubt for the same reasons.

Butter

If a natural food store carries butter, it will be distinguished from commercial butter by the absence of artificial coloring or by the fact that it is produced from raw rather than pasteurized milk. Ordinary butter often contains a yellow dye, yellow #3 to be exact, one of the so-called U.S. Certified Colors. If a manufacturer of natural butter chooses to use a coloring agent it will usually be carotene or annatto bean, neither of which have been shown to be harmful, even to rats.

Like raw cheese, raw milk butter has been subjected to a certain amount of heat during production, so it is not a truly raw product.

Yogurt

Once known best as a 47-point Scrabble word, yogurt has become a household staple, and U.S. consumption is now at three pounds per person per year, with $500 million in annual sales. This is primarily due to the acceptance of yogurt as a low calorie lunch, and it is reasonably low in calories providing you don't pile too much sweet stuff on it.

Commercial yogurts sold in supermarkets often contain chemical emulsifiers and stabilizers, artificial colors and flavors, and white sugar. On the other hand, the natural food versions, which are appearing more frequently in supermarkets as well as natural food stores, use certain plant derivatives, such as guar gum, carob bean gum, gum tragacanth, and irish moss (carrageenan), as thickeners, stabilizers, and emulsifiers. Also, natural sources of color, such as annatto bean, tumeric, and red beet juice, will be employed.

Actually, none of this sounds all that appealing to me in spite of all the "natural" overtones, and I would much prefer to make my own yogurt and control the ingredients. Yogurt making is simple and economical and the initial investment in equipment can range from nothing up to $15 or $20, depending upon how much convenience and perfection you require.

Dairy Products, Eggs, and Substitutes

The first yogurt was probably made quite by accident, in a saddle bag made of some animal's stomach and slung over a camel in the hot sun. Milk kept in the bag curdled and was cultured by the enzymes from the interior lining of the bag. Now, I doubt that you'd care to make your lunch in some smelly old saddlebag, but home yogurt making is basically just that simple. All you really need to do is heat milk to just below the boiling point, add a culture, and keep it at about 115° F for four hours or more. Let's look at this more closely.

a) *The milk:* use any kind you like—cow, goat, sheep, yak, whatever. Whole milk or part skim works best; it is difficult to use 100 percent skim milk. If you want a thick yogurt, add about ⅓ cup of non-instant, nonfat milk powder for each quart of milk. This should be stirred in while the milk is heating, or it may be combined in advance by using a blender.

b) *The heat:* heat your milk to just below the boiling point (smoking not bubbling), and turn off the heat.

c) *The culture:* buy a package of yogurt culture or a small container of plain yogurt from the store. Yogurt culture costs a couple of dollars, but you don't have to buy it everytime you make yogurt. Just add a spoonful or two of your last batch to the new one and the culture perpetuates itself. This process will not go on indefinitely, however, and eventually you must introduce a new culture. You may also buy a small container of plain yogurt and use a spoonful or two of that as your culture. Be sure to find out, however, if the yogurt contains a live culture. If it was pasteurized *after* the culture was added, the culture is no longer viable. This is often the case in ordinary market brands, since pasteurizing the culture makes for a longer shelf life and more consistent taste.

d) *The incubation period:* now that you've got your milk and culture together, the only task remaining is keeping it at a constant temperature for a given period. This is the point at which you can decide to get fancy (read: spend money), or remain simple. All you really need to do is keep it at roughly 115° F. You can use a thermometer to determine when it has cooled to this temperature, or just your sense of touch—115° F feels like lukewarm water, the kind of water that would give you a good shower, but not a great shower. Keeping it at 115° F can be accomplished in an ordinary oven. Often a gas oven with a pilot light is warm enough, or you can preheat a gas or electric oven to 200° F and then turn it off. It should maintain a good temperature for a number of hours. I have even made yogurt in the trunk of a car on a hot day.

On the other hand, if you're the kind of person who wants more security in your life, you can purchase a yogurt maker. These devices are designed merely to keep your milk at a specified temperature for as long as you keep them plugged in. Some make several quarts of yogurt at once, but the average home model makes six or eight little 8-ounce jelly glasses at a time.

How long to culture yogurt is a question of taste. The longer you leave it in your "incubator," the more tart and acidic the taste. Four hours is probably about the minimum time you'd want to culture it, and after ten or so it will be getting pretty sharp. Some fancy yogurt makers even come with automatic timers.

Kefir

Kefir is essentially liquid yogurt, a thick, cultured milk much like buttermilk, usually flavored and sweetened with honey, fructose, and fruit concentrates. I have never seen a supermarket brand of kefir, so there's no comparison to be made. Most kefirs are pretty much the same, although the sweetener may vary, and they may be made with raw milk. However, raw milk kefir, like cheese and butter, will have been subjected to a certain amount of heat in preparation.

Another interesting product is *kefir cheese*. It is basically a super thick kefir, with the consistency of cream cheese, but with a much better taste—worth trying if you come across it.

Ice Cream

If there ever was a mixed blessing, it is ice cream. There's hardly anyone who doesn't like it, let alone crave it. A well-known marathon winner has said, "Without ice cream, there would be chaos and darkness in the world." Many would secretly agree with his hyperbole. Yet in spite of the near universal acceptance of ice cream as a basic food, it is one of the worst foods on earth from a health standpoint. Ice cream has at least six counts against it. (1) It is *cold*—too cold for the digestive system to handle; from the throat on down it represents a physiological trauma. This coldness causes the food to be moved out of the stomach so quickly it does not have time to benefit from the digestive processes taking place there. (2) It is *high in fat*—45 percent for ordinary ice creams, and 58 percent for rich ones, and most of this is saturated. (3) It is *high in sugar*—fourteen teaspoons of sugar in a pint. Great if you're into tooth decay. (4) It is *high in calories*—a pint will put you at least 1000 calories ahead for the day. Of course, you could work that off by running ten miles, or you could just let it gather around your waistline. (5) It may be a *chemical feast*—commercial ice cream often contains a host of artificial colors and flavors, many of which are used in other industries as cleaners, solvents, and even in shoe polish. Until very recently, none of these were required by law to be listed as ingredients. Federal regulations are changing, at last, and although specific chemicals may not be mentioned, at least you get a vague warning like "contains artificial flavor." (6) The combination of cholesterol, saturated fat, and sugars in ice cream will raise blood cholesterol levels more than those elements would individually, and according to recent medical literature the combination of milk and sugar may produce diabetes.[3]

Although it is not possible to speak of a "healthy ice cream," natural food manufacturers have attempted to at least tone down the impact by using only natural flavors and colors. Honey is usually the chosen sweetener as opposed to white sugar, for whatever that may mean to you. In all, ice cream will probably remain a part of most peoples' lives, but it is definitely on the list of foods to be used sparingly.

In addition to an array of ice creams, in every conceivable flavor, stores offer other frozen desserts, like frozen yogurt, sherbert, and ice milk, as well as a variety of treats such as ice cream sandwiches, popsicles, and little "pies" consisting of a slab of ice cream or frozen yogurt wedged between two cookies. Each of these must be evaluated on its own merits. Three and a half ounces of sherbert, for example, has only 140 calories and is 12 percent fat, while one of those "pies" may hit you with over 400 calories and lots of fat, and you can eat one (or three) pretty fast. As always, it's up to you to determine your dietary goals and how each of these foods relates to them.

Eggs

Although eggs are not really a dairy product, they seem to fit into the category by virtue of their nutritional makeup and common use. One can hardly say "milk, butter, cheese . . ." without adding "and eggs."

It should come as no surprise to you that an egg is potentially a little chicken, but only if that egg has been fertilized. You see, hens will continue to lay eggs as long as they are stimulated by the sight and sounds of a rooster and by daylight. These hens may never come in direct contact with a rooster and therefore no fertilization will occur; yet sterile eggs keep coming, not to be hatched into chickens but rather to be lined up in funny shaped cardboard boxes and eventually found in an egg salad sandwich. All this sounds a bit perverse to some people, and they refuse to eat eggs for that reason. Others avoid eggs for health reasons, as they are a source of exceptionally high fat and cholesterol. On the other hand, eggs are often exalted as the finest protein and Nature's perfect food. That it is a high quality protein in terms of amino acid balance is indisputable, but whether that is really important or worth the price in fat intake is another story.

So what's this business about *fertile* eggs? Is there any reason to believe a fertile egg is any more nutritious than a nonfertile egg? Probably not. A fertile egg should not be significantly different in nutritional value from its unfertilized counterpart, provided the hens that produced them had the same living conditions and food. What may affect nutrition, however, is the environment of the hens, including what and how they are fed. Commercial eggs are produced by hens confined to cramped quarters, maintained on abnormal light cycles, and fed chemicalized food. A more natural way of producing eggs allows the hens to run around the barnyard, consort with roosters, "ground-scratch" for their food, and otherwise eat fresh grain, often organically grown. Whether this technique produces a more healthful egg has not been established, although the rich orange yolk, loaded with carotene, which your body converts to vitamin A, contrasts markedly with the pale yellow, sickly looking yolk of an ordinary mass production egg. The real significance, then, of fertile eggs is not the evidence of fertilization as such but what it suggests about the way in which the hens live.

Another popular item is the brown egg, and although they are cute, there is nothing different about a brown egg other than its color. Hens which lay brown eggs simply have a small gland which colors the shell just before the egg is layed. The color probably has some evolutionary adaptive function like camouflaging the egg from predators, but has no nutritive value. People who pay premium prices for brown eggs are paying for esthetics only.

Since we're into exploding myths, lets talk about raw eggs. Anyone who saw the movie *Rocky* will recall that memorable scene where our hero arises before dawn, cracks about five raw eggs into a glass and wolfs them down, after which he jogs off into the sunrise ready to take on the world, or at least Philadelphia. For some reason raw eggs have become associated with strength and stamina. Weight lifters are real big on milkshakes made with a couple of raw eggs. Unfortunately, there's no nutritional logic to this. A raw egg contains little more nutrition than a cooked one, but it does contain a substance called *avidin* which binds up one of the B-complex vitamins, *biotin*, and renders it unavailable to the body. Biotin is critical for the maintenance of a healthy nervous system, and a regular diet of raw eggs could easily lead to a biotin deficiency, resulting in symptoms like depression, dermatitis, and sleeplessness; not to mention chicken breath.

Finally, a plug for egg whites. If you feel uncomfortable about not having egg protein in your diet, but really don't want the fat and cholesterol, just throw that part away—it's all in the yolk. Egg white contains an ample amount of protein, yet zero fat and cholesterol. Feed the yolks to your dog or cat, their short digestive systems are better able to deal with it.

Pro and Con

Dairy products, and eggs, are a great source of protein, calcium, vitamin A, and certain essential fatty acids. What is not so great is that they are also a source of saturated fats and cholesterol.

Although I don't realistically envision a world without dairy products, I would like to see one where people have learned to respect them for what they are—rich foods to be used in moderation. As with meat, there is nothing nutritional in dairy products you cannot get from other foods easily, and without a degree in biochemistry as some would have us believe. A diet of whole grains, fruits, and vegetables will provide all the protein, calcium, linoleic acid, and vitamin A your body can use without the unnecessary saturated fats and cholesterol. It is for most people, however, a boring diet, at least compared to what they're used to. The addition, then, of dairy products, as an alternative to meat, can often spark it up sufficiently for people to stick with it. Dairy is the transition protein between meat eating and total vegetarianism. Most people never make it all the way, and most really don't have to, so long as they learn to moderate their dairy intake and emphasize the use of low fat alternatives like skim milk, egg whites, and low fat yogurt or cottage cheese.

Providing one uses dairy products that are pure and unadulterated, and limits saturated fat intake by product selection and moderation of quantity, the healthy person need not totally eliminate these foods from his life. Be aware, however, that dairy products are the number one source of allergies in the Western diet, and eggs take second place on that list.

Dairy and Egg Substitutes

For those who choose to limit or eliminate dairy products, the natural food industry has created a world of substitutes, almost all of which are based upon that chameleon of foods, the soybean. Soy margarine for butter, tofu for cheese or eggs, soy milk, soy cheese, soy yogurt and even—can it be true?—soy ice cream.

Chosen primarily because of its high protein content and agricultural abundance in this country, the soybean has become the king of natural foods. Its versatile texture and relatively bland taste lend it to a kaleidoscope of applications as meat substitutes and extenders (see Chapter 17), dairy and egg substitutes, or just plain good food in its own right. Soybeans have been subjected to high level food technology to alter their taste, texture, and even molecular structure, and are showing up in all sorts of processed foods often listed only as "vegetable protein." These are highly processed foods, however; we shall confine ourselves here to those foods most closely approximating the natural source.

Margarine

Margarine may be made from any type of oil: corn, soy, safflower, sunflower, palm, coconut, etc. It is considered a butter substitute, although it may be no better, except that it is not an animal product.

Margarine is produced by the hydrogenation of oil, a process discussed in Chapter 5. Once an oil is hydrogenated and in solid form, it is essentially a saturated fat, like butter, and in that sense the value of the polyunsaturated oil is gone. Melting margarine does not alter its saturated nature. Hydrogenation is a chemical process and is not reversed by heat.

Margarines found in natural food stores differ only in their lack of artificial color and flavor. They are generally colored with carotene to produce a more attractive yellow shade. Some offer added wheat germ oil or lecithin but the bottom line is fat, 100 percent.

Tofu

Ever see those odd looking blocks of white stuff floating in water in a plastic bag or box in the supermarket? They were always surrounded by other strange looking foods—funny looking noodles and dried something-or-other. Unless you happen to be Oriental you most likely hurried by, dismissing it as food for foreigners. And food for foreigners is pretty much what it has been for most of its life on Earth. At least one scholar has suggested that the Chinese civilization could not have existed without soybeans, and most of those beans eventually became tofu. Tofu is now becoming an increasingly popular food in the U.S., mainly because it is the perfect substitute for meat and dairy products due to its superior protein content and relatively low percentage of saturated fat (although it is 53 percent fat, most of it is unsaturated). Tofu, sometimes called soybean curd or simply bean curd is nothing more than soybeans which have been cooked, steamed, coagulated, and pressed into blocks. It is low in calories (72 for a 3½-ounce serving) and high in protein (43 percent).

As a dairy substitute, tofu functions quite well in recipes calling for cheese. Although a slice of tofu taken straight from the block will not compare to a slice of cheddar cheese along with a shiny apple and a glass of red wine, when hidden in sauces and seasonings it is often hard to distinguish. Tofu can be used in casseroles, stuffed peppers or pasta, even on pizzas.

Because of its texture, tofu also makes a good egg substitute in recipes. Try scrambling some with your usual spices and adding some peppers, onions, or tomatoes, and you'll be surprised at the similarity.

If you're the adventurous type, you can make your own tofu at home. You can purchase a tofu-making kit in many natural food stores or kitchen gadget shops, cook up some soybeans, and have a go at it. Most of us, however, will prefer the convenience of buying it ready-made, especially at around 50 cents to $1 a pound.

When you're buying tofu, pay attention to the additives used as firming agents or preservatives. Many market brands use calcium chloride or calcium sulfate, and I would avoid these, since we know so little about them.

A good brand of tofu will come packed in *nigari*, sea water which has been dehydrated and desalinated (water and salt removed). What remains is primarily magnesium chloride plus the other minor salts found in sea water other than common table salt. Some natural food brands use only organically grown soybeans in their tofu, and this may or may not be of importance to you.

Soymilk

Soymilk may be available fresh, frozen, or in powdered form in most natural food stores. It is used as a substitute for cow's milk by those who are unable to digest milk or simply wish to avoid or limit dairy products. Many soy infant formulas are being used successfully for babies allergic to dairy milk or by those who have chosen to raise their children as strict vegetarians. The following is a comparison of soymilk and cow's milk with respect to the major nutrients.

	Soymilk*	Cow's milk
protein	3.4g	3.5g
fat	1.5g	3.5g
carbohydrate	2.2g	4.9g
calcium	21mg	118mg
phosphorus	48mg	93mg
iron	.8mg	trace
thiamine (B1)	.08mg	.03mg
riboflavin (B2)	.03mg	.17mg
niacin	.2mg	.1mg

Source: U.S. Dept. of Agriculture Handbook no. 8
*This is the ordinary product, not specifically formulated for infants. In infant formulas, both calcium and iodine are added, the latter to balance out the goitregenic (tendency to produce goiter) nature of soybeans.

Dairy Products, Eggs, and Substitutes

It's easy to see that soymilk stacks up quite well against the competition. In most respects it is a superior product, lower in fat, and higher in essential nutrients. The lower calcium level is misleading, since calcium balance is tied to phosphorus intake and the lower level of phophorus in soymilk makes the calcium all the more available to the body. Remember that calcium requirements are considerably lower for vegetarians than for meat eaters.

Other Soy "Dairy" Products

As soy products become popular with the mainstream public, more and more varieties are being introduced. We now have soy mayonnaise (without eggs or cream), soy cheese (a sort of hard tofu cake), soy yogurt, and soy ice cream. Soy products of this kind take a bit of getting used to, so don't expect them to be exact taste duplicates of their dairy-based counterparts.

Nut Milk

Take a cup of raw almonds, soak them in water overnight, blend in a blender with some additional water, and you've got almond milk. The same thing can be done with cashews, sunflower seeds, sesame seeds, and virtually any edible nut or seed or combination of them. If the flavor is a bit bland for you, try adding some honey and spices like cinnamon, nutmeg, allspice, vanilla, or carob powder. You may also add bananas to give it more body. But remember, this is a high fat, high calorie drink so use it carefully.

Seed Cheese

Soak a cup of whole pastry wheat in water for a day or so until it shows a lot of bubbles. Pour off the liquid into a container and let it ferment in a warm place for 36 to 72 hours. You will now have an active enzyme capable of acting as a culture. Add two cups of this ferment to one cup of sunflower or sesame seeds and blend. Pour this glop into a glass container, put a towel over the top, and let it stand at 75 to 95° F until it cultures into a "cheese" or "yogurt." If it smells sour, you've done something wrong, so best get rid of it. Possible mistakes might be a not-so-clean blender or container, bad tap water, or bad seeds.

Egg Replacers

Egg replacers were designed to substitute for eggs, but most of the commercial brands I have seen in the supermarket contain dried eggs and milk products. One natural food version (Jolly Joan brand) contains arrowroot flour, potato starch, tapioca flour, modified vegetable gums, and leavening. This would definitely be a preferable alternative. Be aware, however, that this is meant to take the place of eggs *in a recipe*, like for a cake or a casserole, where you need an egg-like substance to hold things together. You're not going to be able to whip up a tasty Spanish omelette or two-over-light from an egg replacer, since it is primarily a baking powder-like product designed to substitute for the raising effect of eggs.

Recipes

Soy Butter

½ pint water　　　　　　　1 pint soy oil
2 Tbsp. soy flour

Mix together water and soy flour. Put in heavy frying pan, boil 5 minutes, or until thickened. Strain into mixing bowl. Pour in soy oil, very slowly, beating constantly.

Yeast Cheese

1 cup nutritional yeast flakes　　　2 cups water
　(brewer's yeast)
⅓ cup whole wheat pastry flour

Mix dry ingredients. Stir in water slowly, using a whisk, making a smooth paste and then thinning with water. Heat, stirring continuously until it thickens and bubbles (like pudding). Let bubble 30 seconds, then remove from heat. For variety add garlic powder, onion powder, or any other herbs or spices you like.

Q. *Don't growing children need more protein and calcium than adults?*

A. A child's rate of growth after he has stopped breast-feeding is gradual compared to that of the nursing period. You will recall that human milk is only 6 percent protein and low in calcium, yet it is the perfect food for infants during this rapid growth stage. I can see no reason why a child would need more protein or calcium in later stages when the demands are considerably less.

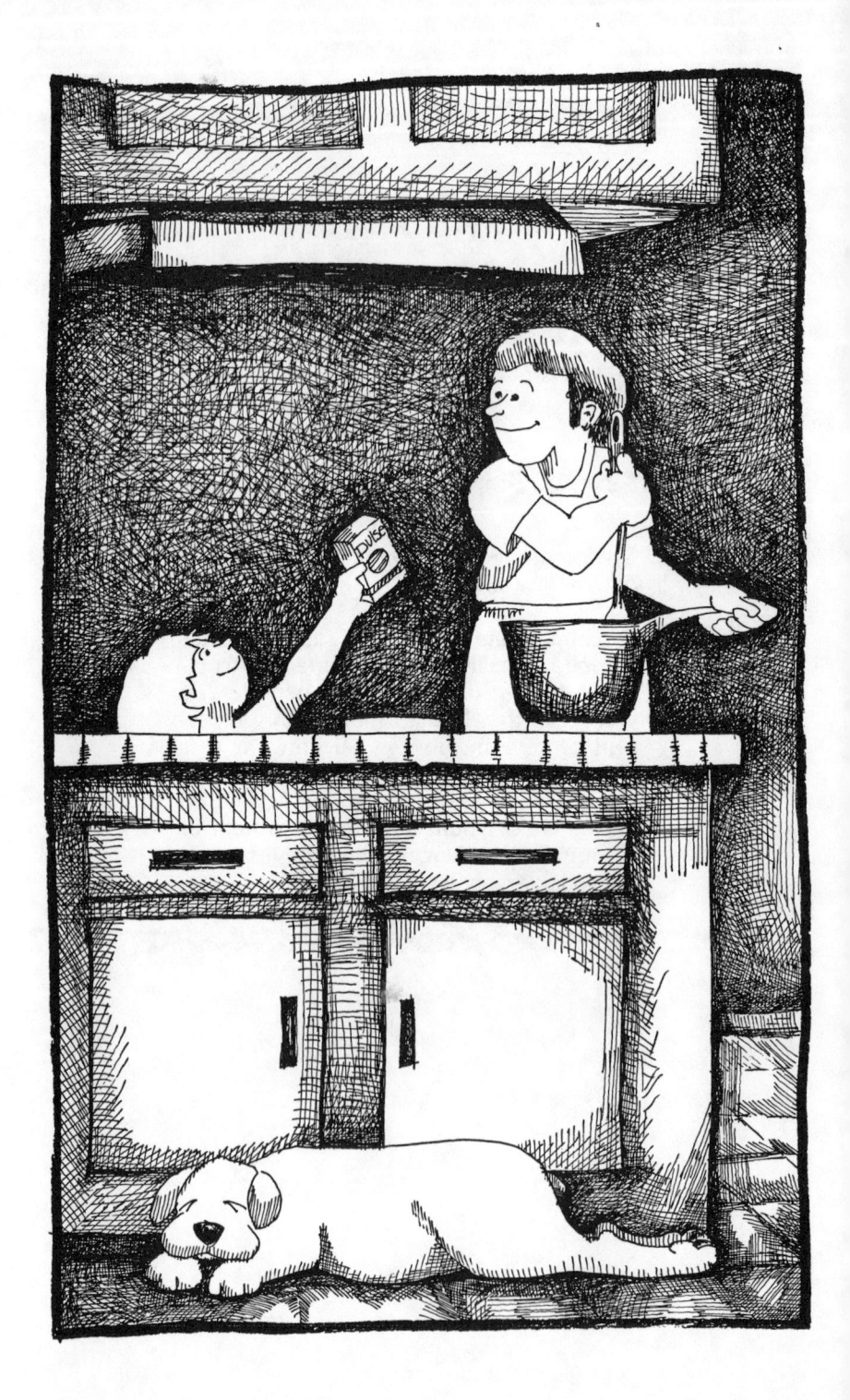

CHAPTER 15

Condiments, Seasonings, Soups, and Seaweed

This chapter is a sort of catch-all for those edibles one finds stacked neatly on shelves in any natural food store and which we use to brighten up our basic foods. Virtually anything you can find in a supermarket in the way of condiments and seasonings may be found in a "natural" version. These products differ from their supermarket sisters in that they are free of chemical additives and white sugar, generally free of hydrogenated fats, and by and large made of higher quality ingredients. In addition, you can often find items designed for people on sodium-restricted or low cholesterol diets.

Mayonnaise

A popular natural food mayonnaise lists the following ingredients: cold-pressed soy oil, eggs, water, honey, lemon juice, seasalt, natural spices. With the exception of that misleading "cold-pressed" business, this appears to be a perfectly acceptable product for those who like to use mayonnaise but prefer not to eat refined sugars and chemical additives. It is, however, a high fat, high cholesterol food and should be treated as such. Most brands will have similar ingredients, some using safflower or other oils instead of soy, but basically the same. You will also find "eggless" mayonnaise, made only with vegetable oil and therefore free of cholesterol. By law, strange as it may seem, these eggless products cannot be called mayonnaise, since that name implies the presence of eggs. They must therefore be labeled "imitation mayonnaise," or some coined term like "vegemaise." Also, commercial spreads called "salad dressings" need not contain eggs, although some do.

Vinegar

Many people drink apple cider vinegar straight from the bottle because they believe it has certain health-giving properties, but none of these claims has ever been substantiated. Vinegar is high in acid, and if you have some reason to want to balance your system with acidity this may be of value. But as far as curing arthritis goes, well that's more a matter of faith than fact.

However, if you just like vinegar on your salad or for marinades, by all means choose one that hasn't been filtered and distilled to death. Apple cider vinegar is the most popular. A good brand will have a gooey strand-like substance floating in it, visible when the bottle is held up to the light. This is known as the "mother" and is supposed to be a sign of purity. At least it is a sign that the vinegar hasn't been filtered too heavily.

Vinegar, incidentally, has a few beneficial topical uses as well. It is an excellent hair rinse which removes leftover soap from the hair and restores the acid PH. Just mix about an ounce in a pint or so of water and pour over your hair after washing out the shampoo. You can then rinse out the vinegar, or leave it in and smell like a salad. It is also pleasing to the skin when added to bath water, restoring the so-called acid mantle, or proper PH of the skin. Sunburn and insect bites both seem to respond well to vinegar.

Salad Dressings

For those who don't care to make their own, an array of pourable salad dressings and dry mixes are available in all possible flavors. Usually based on soy oil, but occasionally on sesame, safflower, and even olive, these dressings are usually free of refined sugar, hydrogenated fats, and additives like polysorbate 80, EDTA, and monosodium glutamate (MSG). But as always, read your labels; you never know what may be sneaking in.

Dry Seasonings

As many natural foods, particularly grains and beans, are rather bland, seasonings play an important role in palatability.

Condiments, Seasonings, Soups and Seaweed

Those skilled in the use of herbs and spices can do wonders with rice and beans, but for those of us who don't know sage from Shinola the industry has created lots of things you can just shake onto your salads, sandwiches, or rice and beans. The most famous among these are Spike, Vegit, Vege-sal, and Dr. Bronner's Mineral Salt and Protein Seasoning. Each of these has different ingredients, usually including various natural mineral salts, dehydrated vegetables, dried herbs and spices, and good old salt itself, unless it specifies otherwise. Both Vegit and Jensen's Broth and Seasoning are excellent low sodium seasonings. You will also see a product called Salt Substitute which is largely potassium chloride, but notice that the bottle bears a warning to consult a physician before using, since excess potassium may be undesirable for persons with kidney problems or certain other conditions.

Liquid Seasonings

From the Oriental cultures have come three closely related liquid seasonings: *shoyu, soy sauce,* and *tamari*. Traditionally, natural shoyu is made from roasted soybeans and wheat, with added water and salt, all carefully fermented and aged to produce a rich black seasoning to put a little spice in your rice. Commercial shoyu is made from defatted soymeal, and the fermentation process is artifically accelerated by temperature control. It may also contain preservatives and other additives. Soysauce is not fermented and is instead produced by a chemical process; it also has artificial color and a preservative like sodium benzoate added, and usually monosodium glutamate.

Tamari, officially, is suppose to be the liquid which forms on the top of miso as it ferments. However, at the moment most of the tamari available in the U.S. is mislabeled and is in fact natural shoyu. This situation is slowly being corrected as true "tamari" begins to appear on the market.

Tamari, or natural shoyu for that matter, has a delicious and mellow taste and is excellent on rice, beans, in salad dressings, and in many dishes where salt is called for. It does, however, contain quite a bit of salt and would be off limits for those restricting sodium One company, Soken, imports a low sodium tamari they call Gentle Tamari, which has a full flavor and only 500mg of sodium per tablespoonful, as compared to 1200mg of sodium in ordinary soysauce.

Miscellaneous Condiments

Olives, pickles, relish, sauerkraut, mustard, barbeque sauce, pasta sauce, etc. are all available in nonchemicalized forms. Some boast "organic" ingredients and other such enticements, but for the most part they are basic products of good quality. Catsup is an interesting case. If a natural catsup contains no sugar, it cannot legally be called catsup, since the official government definition includes a certain amount of white sugar. So, with typical irony, the sugarless catsup must be termed "imitation catsup," or "table sauce."

Soups

It has been found that some foods packed in cans, especially those containing high acid ingredients like tomatoes, tend to be higher than normal in lead. This is because the lead contained in the can itself is being leached into the food. We all know that lead is a dangerous element, and since we cannot avoid breathing it in our air, we certainly don't want to add it to our diets. Health Valley recently began marketing a line of soups in enamel-coated cans which do not leach any foreign substances into the contents. This is a welcome innovation and it is hoped other companies decide to follow Health Valley's example. These soups, additive-free of course, are available in a wide range of flavors, and in both regular and salt-free versions.

Packaged soup mixes are also made for the natural food consumer, but some of these contain raw sugar, so read the labels if this is important to you.

Miso

The growth of interest in the macrobiotic diet has made certain Japanese foods quite popular in the natural food industry. Of these, *miso* is the centerpoint. Made from fermented soybeans, seasalt, and a grain, like barley or brown rice, miso is a black paste which has a multitude of uses in sauces, dressings, and as a soup base. Besides having an excellent taste, it is high in enzymes believed to be valuable to the digestive system, and is considered a natural nonanimal source of vitamin B12. Lots of additional claims have been made for the powers of miso. These range from curing a hangover to protecting against the effects of nuclear fallout. And as bizarre as the latter may seem, it is the result of some serious research by Japanese scientists who have isolated a substance in miso called *zybiocolin*, which has the ability to bind up radioactive elements like strontium 90 and move them out of the body through normal eliminative channels.[1]

If you're too busy to worry about a nuclear war right now and just want a good meal, miso does fine as plain good food. It is, however, quite high in salt, and that should be a consideration for most of us, the relationship between salt intake and hypertension having been well established.

Since miso contains living micro-organisms which may be beneficial, miso afficionados recommend adding it to cooked dishes only *after* they have been taken off the heat. Otherwise you will destroy these elements.

Seaweed

Oh no, now we have to eat seaweed? Surprisingly, seaweed, or more properly sea vegetables, are decidedly on the rise in popularity in the U.S., again due to new interest in Japanese foods among natural food buffs. The more common sea vegetables sold now include dulse, kombu, nori, wakame, hijiki, arame, and agar-agar. Most of these are used in soups and stews for both bulk and seasoning. Dulse, an exceptionally good source of iron, can be rinsed and eaten raw in salads.[2] Nori is rolled into flat sheets and wrapped around rice and other foods, making a popular Japanese snack called *sushi*. Agar-agar is a carbohydrate produced from certain seaweeds. It is used as a substitute for animal gelatin in cooking or in sweets.

Storage

As we have said repeatedly, anything containing oils ought to be a serious candidate for space in your refrigerator, particularly if it is without preservatives. For that reason it is highly recommended that any mayonnaise or salad dressings be kept cold immediately after opening.

Vinegar is its own preservative and need not be refrigerated. Miso, tamari, and dried seaweeds may all be kept safely in the cupboard. In humid climates, seasonings like Spike will attract moisture and stick into a big useless lump. Refrigeration may help retard this process, but the old restaurant trick of adding a little rice as a dessicant is always handy.

Recipes

Just to show you it's possible, here are a couple of oil-free and salt-free salad dressings.

Russian Dressing*

¾ cup cider vinegar
¾ cup water
2 Tbsp. lemon juice
1 Tbsp. chopped onion

1 tsp. dry mustard
1 tsp. garlic powder
⅛ tsp. ground pepper
½ tsp. ground paprika

Combine and mix well.

Vegie-Salad Dressing[5]

1 green pepper
5 tomatoes
1 carrot
1 cucumber (peeled)
3 green onions
1 clove garlic

⅛ cup lemon juice
1 tsp. pure vegetable seasoning
1 bunch parsley
½ tsp. marjoram
1 tsp. basil

Chop vegetables, blend in blender until smooth. Add lemon juice and spices. Add water if needed to get right consistency. Keep refrigerated.

Q. *How does exercise fit into the relationship between diet and health?*

A. Moderate aerobic exercise is definitely beneficial to the body in a number of ways, and I would suggest that without some form of activity like walking or jogging one cannot expect to reap the full benefits of a good diet. This type of exercise increases HDL (see note no. 8, Chapter 1) and may therefore help to slow the rate of atherosclerotic development. It also strengthens the heart muscles, increases circulation and oxygen uptake, aids digestion and elimination, and favorably affects the metabolic rate, resulting in better weight control. It *will not*, however, offer immunity from heart disease, a promise often made in runner's magazines, and there is no reason to believe it will give you any protection from the overall effects of a poor diet. Don't be swayed by the testimonials of world class athletes concerning their junk food binges. These are very special, highly trained individuals in the prime of their lives, and just because they can eat pizza and hot dogs and win marathons doesn't mean they're not doing incalculable harm to their body systems.

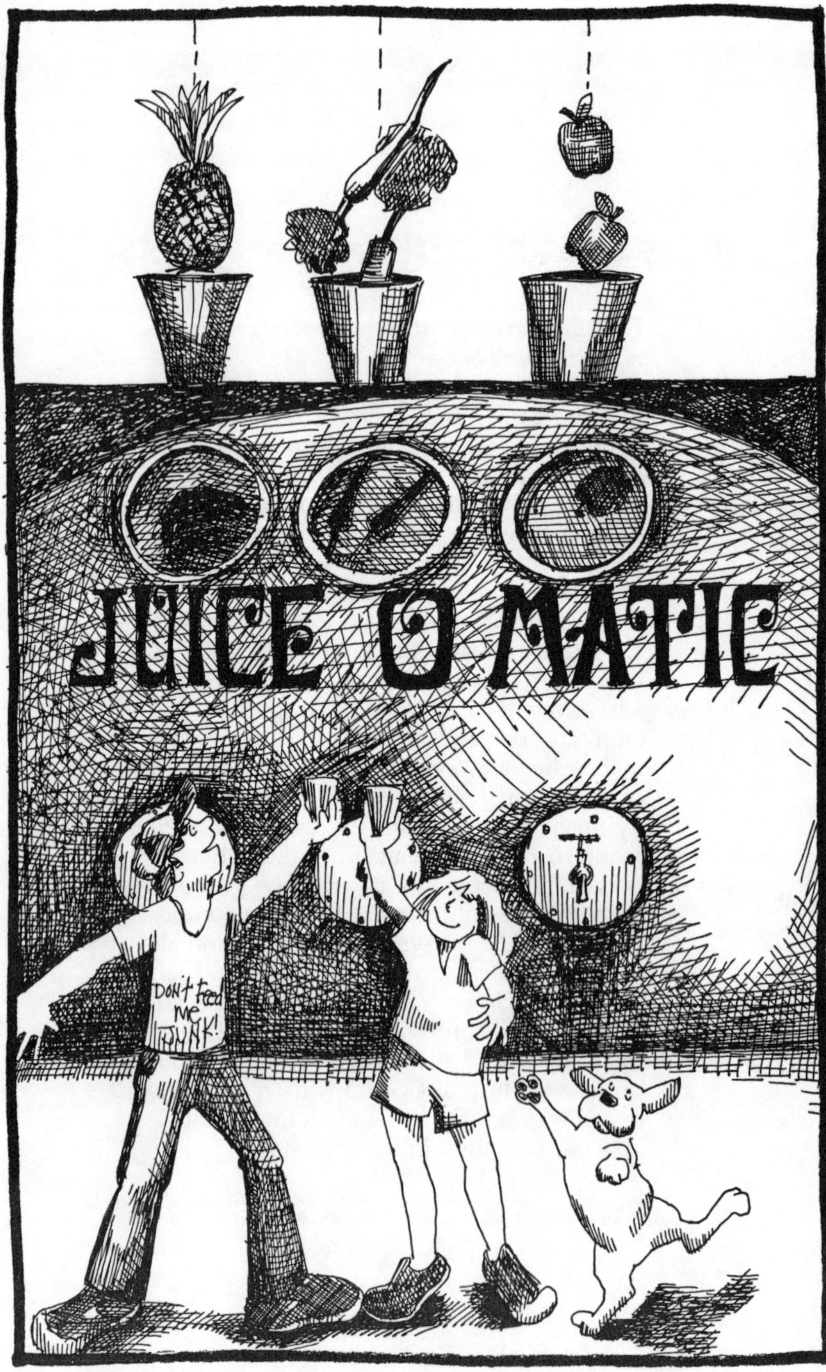
JUICE O MATIC
DON'T feed me JUNK!

CHAPTER 16

Juice and Other Drinks

The juice department at any natural food store leaps out at the customer with an eye-pleasing expanse of color—from bright orange papaya juice to deep purple concord grape. And there are all those tempting blends—apricot-coconut, apple-boysenberry, banana-strawberry. Hardly anyone can get out of the store without taking at least one bottle of juice along. Just how good for you are juices? To answer we need to know a little about how juices are produced and what may or may not be added to them.

It all begins with fruit, but generally not the fruit you see in the market. Those perfectly shaped, shiny red apples will never see the inside of a glass bottle. Most juice producers use "seconds"—fruit which is perhaps undersized, odd-shaped, or otherwise not cosmetically pleasing enough to make the big time at Safeway. None of these characteristics, however, detracts from the fruit's basic goodness. An ugly apple is as nutritious as any beauty you'd pay a dollar for at a mid-city fruit stand. Producers may also buy leftovers from the supermarkets—fruit that has been rejected by customer after customer until it is finally removed from competition. Again, this fruit will produce as fine a juice as any would, and none of this information is meant to imply the consumer is being short-changed in any way. Not all juices are made from reject fruit, by the way; often large companies contract in advance to buy an entire season's crop from an orchard, taking the good, the bad, and the ugly.

Once the fruit has been selected, it is pressed into juice and filtered. The degree of this filtration determines to some extent the nutritional quality of the final product. All juices are filtered somewhat, otherwise you would see stems, leaves, and cores floating around in the bottle, but too much filtering removes essential nutrients. That crystal clear apple juice you see on grocery store shelves has had some of its minerals removed by an ion-resin exchange process. This is done purely in the interest of appearance, the manufacturer being convinced the average shopper is put off by "discoloration." A more legitimate apple juice is murky and cloudy and the bottom of the bottle looks like the Mississippi River.

Fruit Juice

Raw or Pasteurized?

Although it will ordinarily not be stated on the label, all juices found on open unrefrigerated shelves have been pasteurized. Any unpasteurized juice would spoil in a week or two, even under refrigeration, and for large manufacturers this would hardly be enough time to get it to the distributors. Pasteurization involves heat up to 190° F and no doubt has some destructive effects on the juice, resulting in the partial loss of heat sensitive vitamins. This is unfortunate, but without pasteurization, we would have little of the juice available to us today.

Some stores feature raw, unpasteurized juices. These are either made on the premises or by a small local juice producer delivering weekly. These juices, usually in polyethylene bottles, are always kept under refrigeration. Raw juices are expensive, often 50 to 75 percent higher than pasteurized, and this is due partly to high labor costs in the absence of sophisticated automated machinery, and partly to spoilage. You see, when the expiration date on the juice has passed and no one will buy it, it must be dumped. That loss becomes an operating expense and must be figured into the retail cost of the product either by the shopkeeper or the producer, whoever assumes that loss.

Nutritionally, raw juices are always superior, having all their basic nutrients intact. If you value the benefits of fresh raw juice, you might consider investing in your own juicer—it would probably pay for itself in a year.

Fruit Tree or Laboratory?

Whether you buy your juices raw or pasteurized, the variety offered seems limitless. As juices continue to increase in popularity, more and more exotic blends appear on the market. The original blends were based on apple juice with another fruit juice added: apricot, peach, boysenberry, strawberry, grape, cranberry, pomegranate, banana, and so on. As blends become more complicated, the use of pressed fruit juice has given way to *purees* and *concentrates*. A puree is made by reducing the fruit to a pulp and straining out the seeds and skin. A concentrate is a juice that has had most of the water removed through heating or freezing. These have great advantages for the producer: they can be shipped and handled much more efficiently and inexpensively.

Some questions arise, however, as to the purity of these products. If in fact the puree or concentrate is nothing more than fruit that has been pulped or dehydrated, then there is no problem. On the other hand, food technologists have ways of doing things in their laboratories that can mimmick natural foods almost beyond detection. *Whole Foods* magazine reported (April 1978): "One executive of a natural fruit juice company told, with grim humor, of 50 drums of concord grape concentrate which entered a Los Angeles flavor fabricating plant and emerged as 500 drums of concord grape concentrate, which were purchased by an unsuspecting juice bottler."

The important point here is that unless a manufacturer-bottler knows exactly where his ingredients are coming from and can trace them from the farm to the factory, he is as much at the mercy of the unscrupulous as we are as consumers.

The use of concentrates and the dubious nature of their origin brings into focus another area of possible deception. Apple juice may be nothing more than squeezed and strained apples put in a bottle, but it could also be made up of apple concentrate, apple peel, water, and added enzymes. None of this is required to be stated on the label, and the concoction goes on the shelf as "apple juice," just like the genuine article next to it. Of course, the manufacturer using a concentrate will have lower operating costs and hence be able to market his product at a lower cost. Keep that in mind the next time you think you're getting a "deal" on some natural apple juice at the supermarket.

A concerned natural juice producer will go out of his way to make statements on his label that attest to the authenticity of his product even though he is not required to do so by law. Phrases like "made from sound ripe apples" or "no concentrates used" at least put him on the line legally if there were any fraud involved. Personally, I appreciate a manufacturer who puts all the information out front, not just what the courts force him to.

Nectar

When a fruit juice becomes sufficiently depersonalized by the addition of water, sweeteners, and acidifiers, it ceases to be a fruit juice in the eyes of the Food and Drug Administration and is instead a "nectar." By their definition a nectar contains fruit juice and pulp, water, sweeteners like sugar and corn syrup, and optional acidifiers like citric acid, ascorbic acid, and tartaric acid. None of this need be stated on the label, the word "nectar" being sufficient. Sufficient for whom? Sufficient for the FDA, I suppose—they know what's in it; but what about us?

Vegetable Juice

Though fruit juice is by far the runaway best seller, interest in vegetable juices is growing. Tomato juice (the tomato is actually a fruit, but most think of it as a vegetable), of course, has been around at least as long as the Bloody Mary, and carrot juice is making a strong showing of late. Vegetable juices are best when they are fresh and raw. Canned and bottled are available, but their nutritional value is doubtful. Twenty minutes after a vegetable juice is made it begins losing vitamins to air, light, and heat. The true vegie juice fanatic has his own juicer—and a big refrigerator.

Carrot juice is the base for most vegetable juice blends: carrot-celery, carrot-beet, carrot-cabbage, carrot-cucumber, carrot-parsley, and just about every other combination a computer could come up with. There are books that expound on the healing properties of various juice combinations, and you can simply look up your ailment and find a concoction to save you. None of this has been subjected to scientific scrutiny, so it is all a matter of trust at this point. Which is not to say juice won't be helpful in many cases. Vegetable juices are powerhouses of key vitamins, and minerals and many human ailments can be traced to deficiencies of these. Carrot juice is exceptionally high in carotene, which your body converts to vitamin A, and anyone suffering from vitamin A deficiency-related maladies, like poor night vision, will certainly benefit from drinking carrot juice. That's why you never see rabbits carrying flashlights.

One final note on carrot juice. If you drink too much of it you'll turn orange. Seriously, the condition even has a name—hypercarotenemia—an overdose of carotene. The color usually appears in the eyes and on the skin, particularly the palms, where the change is most obvious. The condition is harmless, just funny looking. It should be noted here that there *is* a danger of getting too much vitamin A from animal foods (e.g. liver). But the "vitamin A" found in plant foods is in a preformed state and is only converted by the body into vitamin A as needed; and therefore no danger exists from these sources.

Thoughts on Juice

Is juice a natural food? Probably not in the strict sense, since even a raw juice lacks much of the fiber present in the fruit it came from, and pasteurized juices have had nutrients destroyed. Nevertheless, pure juice is close enough to the source to be acceptable, especially if the alternative is Coke or Pepsi. People with blood sugar problems should be aware that fruit juices produce that rapid elevation in blood sugar followed by the typical hypoglycemic "low." In the normal person moderate amounts of fruit juice (a glass or two a day) should have no deleterious effects, but people drinking a quart or more a day of juice may be asking for the sugar blues.

The question of pesticide residues comes up when we think of juices. If the fruit is heavily sprayed, like pineapples for example, does the pesticide make its way into the juice? Chances are pretty good that it does, and the purist may seek to avoid juices from heavily sprayed crops or look for reputable organic juices. In states like California, where there is government regulation of organic growers, if juices are produced within the state and labeled as being from organically grown fruit, it is a fair assumption that the article is genuine. If no such laws or monitoring exist, you take your chances.

As mentioned in the preceding chapter, foods high in acid tend to leach metals like lead out of the insides of cans, especially if they are lead soldered cans. Since fruit and vegetable juices like tomato, orange, grapefruit, and pineapple are quite acidic, they may very well contain more than you've bargained for.

Soft Drinks

The ongoing campaign by the natural foods industry to bring more and more mainstream shoppers into natural food stores or, even better, to bring more natural foods into the major supermarkets has spurred the development of many "alternative" products. The philosophy is simple: find out what people like (translation: what they are buying), and try to duplicate it using only natural ingredients, or close enough to natural to pass. Obviously, Americans drink a lot of soft drinks, and commercial soda pop is not exactly a fountain of health. Cola drinks may contain caffeine (which overstimulates certain glands), phosphoric acid (which can take the enamel off your teeth), caramel (a suspected mutagen), and sugar—lots of sugar. The Coca-Cola company, for example, buys 10 percent of all the sugar consumed in the U.S., and each 12-ounce can of your favorite cola contains seven teaspoons of sugar.

Natural foods companies have tried to eliminate some of the more objectionable components of these soft drinks and still produce a palatable product. They will taste different, no doubt, and you'll never fool a kid into thinking it's Coke once he's had The Real Thing, but tastes are mutable, and sooner or later you adjust to everything in life.

So, what do we have? We have colas, root beers, lemon-limes, and every conceivable fruit flavor—even some herb-based drinks with ginseng in them. These contain no caffeine, no phosphoric acid, no caramel, and no white sugar. What they do contain is filtered, carbonated water, some kind of sweetener (usually honey or fructose), and various natural spices and oils—oil of lemon, oil of sweet birch, anise, cloves, cassia, vanilla, etc. Lemon or lime flavors also have added citric acid for that thirst-quenching tang. Except for the sugars, this is not all that bad, although I wouldn't recommend a gallon a day. A cheaper and far more nutritious way to make soda for you and your kids is to simply mix natural fruit juice with a carbonated mineral water like Calistoga or Perrier.

Water

To the person with no awareness whatsoever of the relationship between what you are and what you eat, the buying and drinking of bottled water seems patently absurd. Why spend good money on water when all you have to do is turn on the faucet and out it comes? If only water came out of that tap, I'd be the first to applaud their insight. Unfortunately, tap water is fast becoming one of the most untrustworthy of our household resources. Depending on the area in which you live, your drinking water may be "acceptable" (by government standards), questionable, or downright dangerous. The air is usually just as bad, but the water we can at least control on a personal level.

Your tap water probably contains chlorine, possibly fluorine, and in an alarming number of instances, carcinogenic, mutagenic, and teratogenic chemicals (mutagens can increase the incidence of genetic mutations; teratogens, birth defects) that have found their way into your water system courtesy of local industry. There are many who believe that Love Canal is the tip of the proverbial iceberg. In addition, even water protected from all of these assaults inevitably contains concentrations of heavy metals, like cadmium and copper, leached from the very pipes carrying it to your house.

Many people have decided that drinking from the tap just isn't worth the risk anymore, and have turned to various sources of bottled water. They may have a local company that delivers spring water, purified water, or distilled water to them in 5-gallon bottles, or they may buy their gallon jugs through supermarkets and natural food stores. Outside major supermarkets, in many areas of the country are water-dispensing machines you put a dime or so in and fill up your jug. It's a sign of the times, and a prediction—we may all have no choice in the future.

Let's look at the different types of potable water available. Spring water or mineral water is supposed to be drawn from a naturally occurring artesian well known to be safe from pollution, and bottled without further treatment. Purified water is just tap water that has been run through filters to remove various impurities, including large particles and gases like chlorine. Purified water, however, will still contain heavy metals from pipes. Distilled water is 100 percent water—just hydrogen and oxygen, but only if in addition to being distilled it has been filtered through a column of activated charcoal to remove chlorine and other gases which would survive the distillation process.

Deception is not unheard of in the water business, and you would be wise to deal with a large, well-established bottler and avoid "bargains." An investigation in California in the early 1970s found a number of bottled waters to be straight from the tap.

Mineral vs. Distilled Water

After looking carefully at the situation, you've made your decision for mineral water or distilled water and are pleased with your progressive thinking. All of a sudden some health "expert" comes along and says "Don't drink distilled water, you'll leach all the minerals out of your body!" or "Don't drink mineral water, you'll give yourself arthritis!" Oh no, what now? Controversy rages, as much as it can really rage in the face of no evidence, over the relative merits of mineral versus distilled water. Some say mineral water is too high in certain salts and will aggravate your joints, and besides it can't be trusted anyway since you never know what's getting into those artesian wells. Others say distilled water, due to its lack of minerals, will cause your body to give up its stored minerals to achieve a balance, and this results in critical losses of these essential elements. Neither theory should be cause for any great concern. The amount of essential minerals taken in drinking water is miniscule compared to that you get from fruits and vegetables, and your natural food diet should provide you with an abundance of minerals such that any leaching that may go on would be irrelevant to your health. I prefer distilled water since I'm 100 percent certain it's pure. I have my own distiller, so I don't have to rely on anyone else's integrity (see Chapter 20 for information on distillers).

One major advantage to producing your own drinking water or having it delivered is that the gallon jugs you buy in the market are usually made of plastic. I've never had the water analyzed, but the smell and taste of the plastic in the water made me very suspicious about what evil things might be getting into the water. If possible, try to get your water in glass.

Carbonated Water

Occasionally one likes the taste and feel of a carbonated drink, but doesn't want the calories of a soda or beer. Since everyone seems to be on some kind of reducing diet these days, no-calorie drinks have gotten very popular. Some, like Perrier, have even achieved a certain social status, and one is afraid to drink it without being properly attired.

These drinks are usually valid mineral waters from valid unpolluted wells, and quite distinct from ordinary club soda, which is generally just tap water that has been artificially carbonated. Carbonated waters have one drawback, they're expensive, too expensive for most people to use as their sole source of drinking water. If you're rich you can drink it all day, or even fill your hot tub with it if you like.

Selection and Storage

If you're concerned with purity in a juice, look for one made without concentrates, only fresh juice or pure purees. If you're concerned about pesticides, look for organic juice produced in a state where the word "organic" on the label has a legal definition. Knudsen and Westbrae are two reliable brands in California. If you're concerned about calories or too much sugar, watch out for added sugars, extra concentrates, and nectars. And if you're concerned about fat, by all means don't choose a juice with coconut in it. Coconut is almost totally saturated fat and will raise your cholesterol level as much as a hamburger.

Once juice is opened, it should be refrigerated, as yeasts in the air will cause it to spoil. Before opening, a pasteurized juice should be kept out of direct sunlight. A raw juice should always be refrigerated. Sodas are rather resistant to spoilage due to the added acids, which deter oxidation, but should be refrigerated after opening. Water requires no special storage conditions.

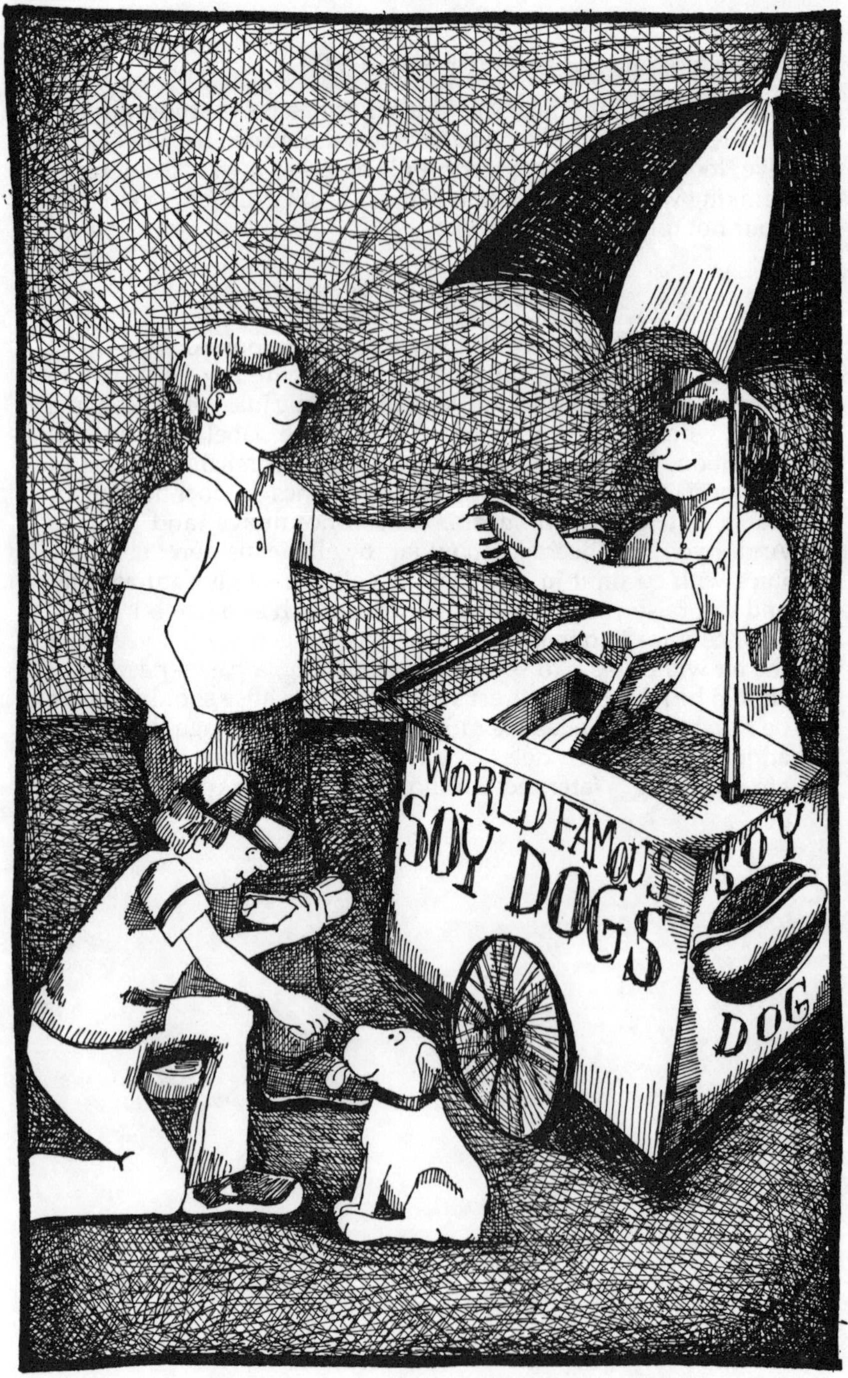

WORLD FAMOUS
SOY DOGS
SOY
DOG

CHAPTER 17

Meat and Meat Substitutes

The arguments for and against eating meat go on and on, forcing anyone aware of them to take a hard look at his priorities. Many have decided to eliminate meat entirely, while others enjoy meat and seek only to moderate its use. For the latter group, the industry has created a full array of meats that at least are free of major contaminants.

Frozen meats, including bologna, salami, wieners, bacon, sausage, ground beef, and even liver, derived from animals that have not been fed or injected with growth hormones, and containing no nitrates or nitrites, artificial colorings, or preservatives are now widely available. The relationship between nitrites and cancer is highly suspect and so is that between hormones like DES and vaginal cancer in daughters, so this appears to be at least a prudent approach to meat eating. Needless to say, the intrinsic problems with meat, i.e., saturated fats, cholesterol, and lack of fiber, continue to exist.

Processed meats, like luncheon meats and hot dogs, will be found in the frozen food sections of many natural food stores. Since they contain no preservatives, freezing is the only way to protect them against deterioration. You can expect these products to cost considerably more than those which are chemically preserved and therefore require no freezing or special handling since spoilage problems are minimal.

With the advent of massive supermarket-size natural food stores, entire meat departments, with banks of glass display coolers and white-aproned butchers have appeared, featuring fresh meat, fish, and poultry all raised by natural means. In addition to the absence of chemical additives, this often means that the animals were allowed to roam and graze, instead of being force-fed in a pen, and were raised on natural foods. As these meats become more and more popular, production will increase, and prices will drop. In some areas prices already compete with those of commercial supermarket meats.

Meat Substitutes

Many people are willing to give up meat to improve their health, but are not yet prepared to live on rice and beans. They like the taste of meat, the texture of meat, and dishes made with meat. The idea of a bowl of chili without meat or something that tastes like meat is, for this person, inconceivable. What shall we do without meat?

Once again, it is the venerable soybean to the rescue. Because the person who enjoys meat is by no means unusual, an entire industry has developed to meet his needs. Meet the *soycrafters*. These are companies that develop and produce *meat analogs*, products which taste like meat and feel like meat, but are in fact made only of plant matter, mostly soy. They have taken the soybean into the laboratory, analyzed it, taken it apart, and invented ways of putting it back together that drastically alter its texture. The result is known broadly as *textured vegetable protein* or simply TVP. "TVP" is actually a trademark owned by Archer Daniel Midland Company, so, although the expression has become widely used as a general name for such products, we will use the abbreviation T.V.P. here for convenience in referring to textured vegetable protein products generally and not the trademark TVP.

T.V.P. by itself does not taste like meat, it merely has a texture which is acceptable as a substitute. To produce a taste comparable to meat, flavoring must be added. It would be nice to think that the clever use of herbs, spices, and other natural flavorings could closely imitate the flavors of beef, chicken, and pork, but so far this has not been accomplished, and artificial flavorings must be relied upon. Although you can purchase an unflavored T.V.P. with which you can experiment using your own seasonings, most people prefer the artificially flavored products like beef T.V.P., chicken T.V.P., and ham T.V.P. Bacon bits is another enormously popular T.V.P. product. Again, artificially flavored, they taste remarkably like dried bacon yet contain no animal fats or cholesterol.

What do you do with T.V.P.? Anything you would do with ground meat, actually. Make it into patties or "meat" loaves, put it in stews and soups, in lasagne, tacos, or on pizza. Or use it as an extender to stretch your hamburger or tuna fish salad to meet your budget. Even the Defense Department is doing it. The military is saving $6.2 million a year by adding 20 percent T.V.P. to their ground meat dishes. Creamed chipped T.V.P. on toast, anyone?

For those without the inclination or time to create their own exotic dishes from basic T.V.P., several companies have long produced canned meat analogs in a huge variety of forms and flavors. Worthington Foods and Loma Linda Foods both market products like hot dogs, hamburgers, sausages, chicken parts, beef chunks, etc., all made essentially from textured soy protein. I have seen entire restaurants based on these products; you can sit down and order chicken caccitore or veal parmigiana and never tell it from the real thing. Originally these meat substitutes were made from gluten, the major protein isolated from wheat, and often used by the Chinese. Like textured soy, gluten is a high protein and highly refined product. One problem with gluten is that many people are allergic to it.

Recently, other types of meat alternatives have appeared on the market, many not employing soy protein at all. These products use nuts, seeds, grains, and beans, along with dried vegetables, herbs, spices, and natural flavors, to produce mixtures that can be made into burgers and "meatballs" or used in any type of dish requiring ground meat. They may not taste quite as much like meat as the artificially flavored products, but the texture similarity is usually satisfying enough and they are far healthier. A few worth mentioning are Nature's Burger by Fantastic Foods, Sesame Burger by Fearn, and various falafil mixes by Westbrae, Fantastic Foods, and Sahara.

The frozen food department is another place to look for meat analogs. Everything from soyburgers to TV dinners has been created out of plant products and attractively packaged in ready-to-pop-in-the-oven forms.

If you prefer doing things from scratch, buy some soybeans, cook them up, and create your own soyburgers or whatever. Hardly a natural food cookbook exists that does not have a few recipes to get you started.

Tofu and Tempeh

Two other soy products deserve mention here, not because they taste like meat, but because they act as meat replacers in the sense of providing basic protein, and at a cost far lower than meat.

Tofu we met before as a dairy substitute. It may also serve as a meat substitute and many books, like *The Book of Tofu* (William Shurtleff and Akiko Aoyagi, Ballantine Books, 1979) will show you how to create satisfying meatless meals like tofu burgers, tofu cutlets, and even barbequed tofu.

Tempeh originated in Indonesia and is a cultured or fermented soy product. A mold called *Rhizopus oligosporus* is used to innoculate soybeans which have been split, cooked, and dehulled. The fermenting concoction is then left to stand in a warm place overnight and then is ready to go. Its significance is that during the fermentation process, protein complexes are broken down into more easily digestible forms, and certain B-complex vitamins are increased in potency. It is one of the few non-animal sources of B12, one ounce of tempeh being sufficient to supply the minimum daily requirement for this vitamin. Making tempeh at home on a small scale is quite easy, and instructions are given in the *Farm Vegetarian Cookbook* (ed.: Louise Hagler, The Book Publishing Co., 1978). Natural food stores often sell tempeh kits, including spores, soybeans, and instructions to get you started. The spores must be purchased originally but can be maintained and reproduced at home after that.

Thoughts on Textured Protein

While any food that helps to reduce the national intake of saturated fats and cholesterol is more than welcome, one has to question the "naturalness" of a product which has undergone as much intense processing and restructuring as has textured vegetable protein. Texturizing alters the molecular weight of proteins and affects the way in which they combine with other ingredients. At least one study suggests that the amino acids react with each other to produce derivatives which have had adverse effects on the kidneys of laboratory animals. The substance in this study, however, was not processed at all like the products being used for food, and therefore the test results are not considered strong enough to warrant product withdrawals.

Others feel that vitamins and minerals are destroyed and rendered unavailable by the processing, and there are always the nagging doubts about the safety of artificial flavors. Textured vegetable protein is, however, a complete protein, and despite its possible drawbacks may prove to be one of the most important foods of the future.

Selection and Storage

Luncheon meats without preservatives should be bought frozen and kept frozen until ready to use. Once a package of bologna or hot dogs has been defrosted, it will most likely keep about a week under refrigeration, so it is advisable to defrost only what you'll use in that length of time. *Salmonella* is nothing to fool around with and salmonella loves lunch meats.

Tofu is good for a couple of weeks under refrigeration, but only if the water is changed every few days. When tofu has spoiled it has a distinctly sour taste. Tempeh should be kept refrigerated for a week or so.

T.V.P. is a reasonably stable product and for anything but long term storage, no special environment is necessary.

As always, any vegeburger mixes containing nuts, seeds, or other high oil foods must be considered candidates for rancidity and should be protected accordingly.

Recipes

Beanburgers

2 cups cooked, drained, and mashed beans (pintos, navy beans, great Northern beans, or soybeans are OK)
1 onion, chopped
2 egg whites (or equivalent amount of egg replacer)
1 cup bulgur (also could substitute whole wheat flour, raw rolled oats, wheat germ, cooked rice, etc.)
1 tomato, blended
1 vegetable bouillon cube, softened
½ tsp. garlic powder
½ tsp. parsley flakes
2 Tbsp. salt-reduced tamari
Season to taste.

In large bowl mix all ingredients thoroughly. Spoon ½ cup-size burgers onto oiled baking pan. Cook in 350° oven for 25 minutes on one side. Flip and cook 15 minutes longer. Serve on whole wheat buns or pita bread with your favorite condiments. Makes 8 burgers.

Sloppy Joes (with T.V.P.)[2]

1 large onion, diced
2 medium green peppers, diced
3 Tbsp. oil
1½ cups boiling water
2½ cups tomato sauce
1–2 Tbsp. chili powder

2–3 tsp. salt
1 Tbsp. soy sauce (tamari)
1 Tbsp. mustard
2 Tbsp. honey or molasses
1½ cups dry T.V.P.
½ tsp. pepper

Sauté onion and peppers in oil. Add remaining ingredients. Simmer together for 20 minutes and serve over whole wheat buns.

Italian Nonmeat Balls[1]

1 lb. tofu, mashed well
2 egg whites, lightly beaten
½ cup whole wheat bread crumbs
2 tsp. vegetable bouillon
½ tsp. onion salt
½ tsp. Italian seasoning

½ tsp. garlic powder
3 Tbsp. grated parmesan cheese
1 Tbsp. dry onion flakes
¼ tsp. pepper
⅛ tsp. nutmeg

Mix together and form into balls. Brown in oil. Use with your favorite spaghetti recipe.

Q. *Are there good meat substitutes not based on soy protein?*

A. Meat alternatives have recently appeared on the market — not employing soy protein at all. These products use nuts, seeds, grains, and beans, along with dried vegetables, herbs, spices, and natural flavors, to produce mixtures that can be made into burgers and "meatballs" or used in any type of dish requiring ground meat. They may not taste quite as much like meat as the artificially flavored products, but the texture similarity is usually satisfying enough and they are far healthier. A few worth mentioning are Nature's Burger by Fantastic Foods, Sesame Burger by Fearn, and various falafil mixes by Westbrae, Fantastic Foods, and Sahara.

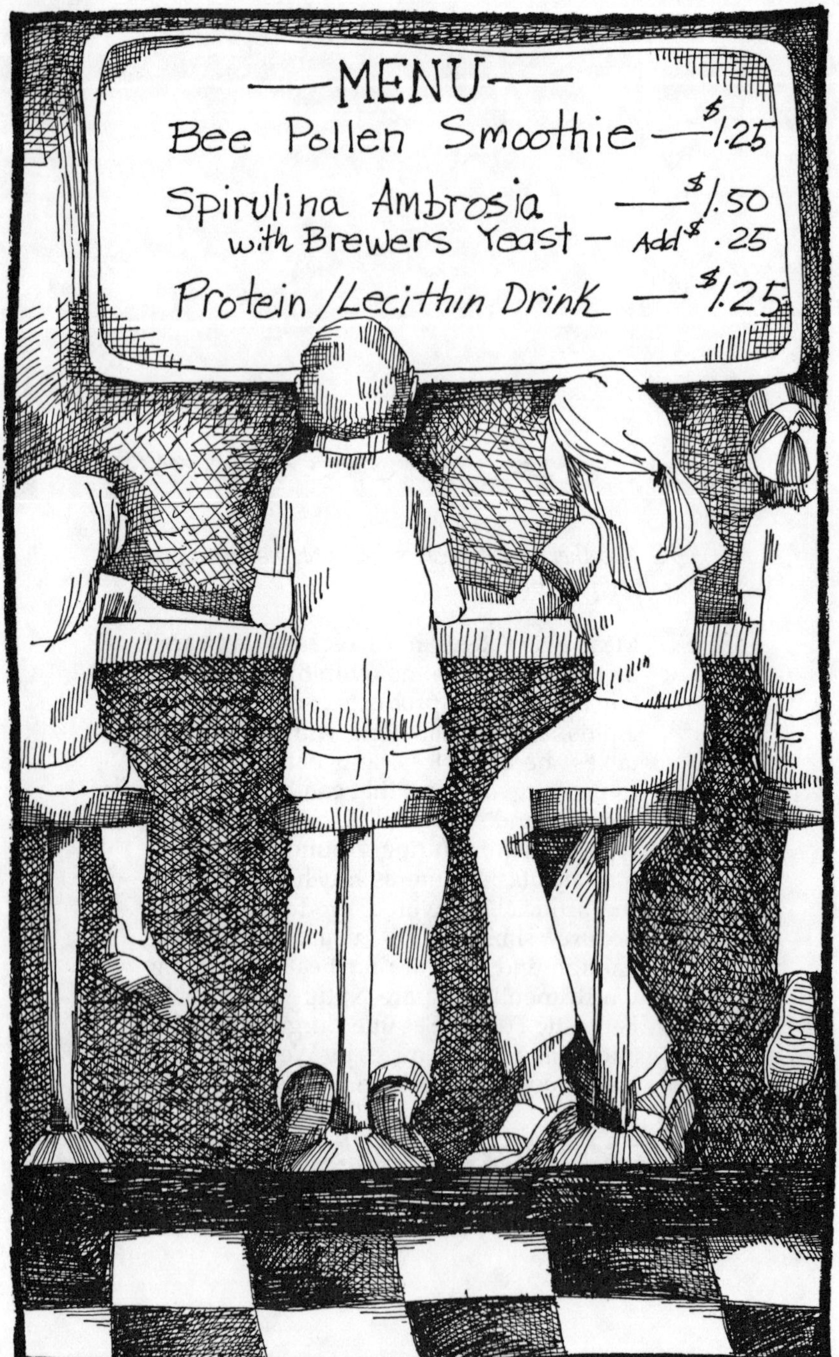
—MENU—
Bee Pollen Smoothie — $1.25
Spirulina Ambrosia — $1.50
with Brewers Yeast — Add $.25
Protein / Lecithin Drink — $1.25

CHAPTER 18
Supplementary Foods

A few foods are so unique that they defy categorization, and so must be thrown together under their own rather nebulous heading. These foods appear to have no use other than as supplements to the diet; some do the job quite well and others are of questionable value.

Lecithin

When soybeans are processed into textured proteins, one phase of the operation involves the removal of a natural substance called lecithin. It is composed of fatty acids, glycerine, phosphoric acid, and choline, and is found in many natural foods. It is also produced quite routinely in the body and is a normal component of human bile. So why would anyone want to supplement their diet with a substance their liver produces for free? The answer to this lies in the fallacy known as "more is better." Many people operate on the notion that if something is good for you, more of it must be even better for you. Although this concept has been proven false at every turn, the attraction persists, and the big attraction to lecithin is its relationship to fat metabolism.

One of the natural functions of lecithin is the breakdown and absorption of fats into the body, owing to its ability to attract both water and oil. This is quite important since several critical vitamins are fat-soluble (A,D,E,K) but must be used in a water-based system. So, the word got out that lecithin breaks down fats. In characteristic fashion, lay nutritionists seeking recognition and the press seeking headlines molded and distorted this information, and now have millions of people believing that taking lecithin will break down the fat stored in your waistline or thighs and miraculously make you skinny without the agony of calorie reduction and exercise. The vitamin industry, of course, was not at all upset by this sudden interest in an otherwise obscure supplement, and lecithin was soon hitting the big time with full-page color ads in national health magazines. It is now one of the biggest sellers in most health food stores.

Sorry to say, but no evidence exists that lecithin will shrink your fat storage centers. Lecithin does have important functions for good health, but the amount necessary is easily provided by a proper diet. Sources of lecithin include egg yolks, liver, brains (yummy!), whole grains, nuts and seeds, and unrefined vegetable oils.

If you still want lecithin, however, plenty of stores will be glad to sell it to you. It is usually available in three forms: liquid, granules, and capsules. The liquid is the most natural and economical form, but has a thick oily texture reminiscent of axle grease, which tends to stick to your tongue and teeth and which many people find unpleasant. Granules have been processed to a greater state of edibility, and can be mixed into drinks or even eaten on salads, although they taste a bit waxy. Capsules are easy to swallow, but the amount of lecithin in each capsule is minimal. The ratio is one tablespoon of liquid equals two tablespoons of granules equals twelve capsules. The laws being what they are, a so-called lecithin capsule may not contain pure lecithin at all, but merely soy oil which has some lecithin naturally occurring in it; yet the label is permitted to read "Lecithin Capsules."

If taking lecithin does you no good, does it do you any harm? Well, it might. Lecithin is, after all, a fat, and more fat in your diet you don't need. It is also high in phosphorus, and foods too high in phosphorus tend to throw off the balance of calcium and magnesium, and the body demands more, which may be leached from the bones. I doubt that one or two lecithin capsules a day would produce anything as dramatic as osteoporosis, but if the "more is better" syndrome prevails, more and more lecithin will be taken. I've met many people who take twelve or more capsules a day. One possible value of lecithin is as a sort of oil "substitute" in recipes. One tablespoon of lecithin may be used to replace up to two-thirds of a cup of oil without significantly affecting the quality of the finished product. This would significantly decrease the amount of fat consumed, always a desirable goal.

Brewer's Yeast

Back in the old days, when beer making was not dominated by chemicals, a by-product of brewing was a yeast which grew in the vats. This yeast was analyzed and revealed to be an excellent source of B-complex vitamins as well as some important trace minerals and proteins. This substance came to be known as brewer's yeast, although today's brewer's yeast has never seen the inside of a brewery. It is produced in laboratories, grown on molasses or whey, spray dried, and packed into drums for shipment to bulk dealers or packagers who put it into cans, bottles, or plastic bags. It is now more properly called *nutritional yeast*, the term "brewer's yeast" being primarily of historical interest.

Nutritionally, brewer's yeast has some strong points and some weak points. It contains a full complement of amino acids, iron, and B vitamins, as well as a few hard-to-get trace elements like selenium and chromium. It is, however, a high phosphorus food and anyone using brewer's yeast regularly should consider some form of calcium supplementation to balance the phosphorus. This can be accomplished by adding calcium lactate or calcium gluconate powder, or a high calcium food like nonfat milk powder. Yeast is also high in *purines*, which produce uric acid, a prime factor in *gout*, a painful disease of the joints. Anyone with a high uric acid level should steer clear of brewer's yeast.

The taste of brewer's yeast is a subject on which you will certainly get a definite opinion, but rarely a consensus. Views run from "it makes me gag" to "you get used to it after a while." Occasionally you will find that maverick who actually likes yeast, but he is the exception. There's no way to describe the taste of yeast. You just have to try it for yourself. Chances are you won't like it the first time, but will eventually come to terms. Some people experience a lot of gas from yeast, but I think that has more to do with what they mix with it rather than the yeast itself. In attempting to disguise the taste, people often mix yeast in fruit juices, and the combination of the acids and sugars in fruit juice with yeast can be unsettling. I always recommend mixing it in water—you can't hide the taste anyway, so you might as well take it straight. Start with a teaspoon or two and work yourself up to two tablespoons a day if you wish to use it at all. Once you've adapted to the taste, and some people even like it immediately, you'll find it useful as a condiment, sprinkled on salads and soups. Some even say it tastes like Parmesan cheese. If you should decide to supplement your diet with yeast, be certain you are getting brewer's yeast or nutritional yeast, not the type of active yeast used for baking, as this will result in severe gastric disturbance.

Bee Pollen

While some bees are out collecting nectar to be stored as honey in the hive, others are picking up tiny granules of plant pollen from the anthers (male sexual elements) of flowers. They pack this dust together into tiny balls that they carry on their hind legs back to the hive to be deposited in the honeycomb, later to be used as a source of protein, vitamins, and minerals during the slow season. Now, a good beekeeper knows that his frugal and foresighted little friends always collect and store much more honey and pollen than they will ever need for their winter season, and so he is able to draw some of this surplus for himself. A pollen-collecting device which obligates the bees to squeeze through a narrow opening is fitted to the hive entrance for a certain time period. As the bee wriggles through this small space, the balls of pollen fall off and are collected below, much to the bee's frustration.

At regular intervals, the beekeeper collects the pollen and stores it under refrigeration. It may be bottled and marketed in this fresh, unprocessed form, heat-dried, freeze-dried, or pressed into tablets. The result is an extremely high quality food, containing all known and probably unknown nutrients— capable of sustaining life itself were you able to get enough calories from it, although it is somewhat high in protein. Problem is, it's darned expensive and out of reach except as a supplement to the diet, unless you're one of those people who puts Perrier in their hot tub.

But, as a supplement, it is without superior. The following is an analysis of one brand:

Supplementary Foods

Fresh Hawaiian Bee Pollen

	Amount in 1 oz
Calories	90
Protein	7.0 grams
Carbohydrate	12.0 grams
Fat	2.0 grams
Sodium	10.0 mg
Fiber	1.5 grams
Vitamin A (Carotene)	100 I.U.**
Vitamin C	1.2 mg
Vitamin B1	0.5 mg
Vitamin B2	0.6 mg
Niacin	3.0 mg
Calcium	100 mg
Iron	1.8 mg
Vitamin B6	0.2 mg
Vitamin B9	0.3 mg
Vitamin B12*	7.0 mcg
Biotin	12 mcg
Pantothenic Acid	0.4 mg
Vitamin E	3 I.U.
Copper	.04 mg
Magnesium	40 mg
Phosphorus	100 mg
Zinc	1.5 mg

*This may be misleading since the typical nutrient analyses done for labeling purposes often reveals "B12 activity," which is not really an assurance that true B12 is present. Further (and more costly) tests are required to detect true vitamin B12.

**International Units.

Source: Label of product called "Fresh Hawaiian Bee Pollen," produced by the Hawaiian Pollen Co., Honolulu, Hawaii.

In addition, it contains 22 amino acids, a host of trace elements, including potassium, aluminum, barium, boron, chromium, manganese, strontium, and more than 80 live enzymes. All this for only 90 calories—truly a food of high nutritional value.

Pollen is the chosen "energy food" of countless long-distance runners, professional athletes, and even Olympic contenders. It has also been claimed to have considerable healing properties, particularly with regard to prostatitis (inflammation of the prostate).

Fresh pollen is the best way to go, and the most costly, although dried pollens are perfectly fine, providing excessive temperatures were not used in the drying process. Pollens are sometimes air-dried or sun-dried, and this should result in no significant loss of nutrients. Those subjected to temperatures above 130° F during either drying or processing into tablet form will have undoubtedly suffered some nutritional losses.

How do you eat it? Pollen has a taste pleasant to most people, sort of like dried honey, and many eat it straight from the package. If the taste doesn't particularly knock you out, you can mix it in juice or sprinkle it on fruit, yogurt, or cereal. An ounce a day is sufficient for the average person seeking a balanced supplement not produced in a vitamin laboratory. Athletes in training often take up to three ounces a day.

Spirulina

As this is being written, a new "superfood" is being introduced to the natural foods market. By the time you read this, spirulina may be an enormously significant food in world nutrition or as obscure as the Edsel. Spirulina is a micro-algae which grows in tropical desert lakes and is harvested and dried into a deep green powder. Nutritionally, it is a remarkable 70 percent protein,[1] highly assimilable, and a good source of vitamin A, B-complex, and many important trace minerals. It is thirty-five times more productive than soybeans, and far higher in protein.

All this sounds wonderful; the only problem is the taste. On a palatability scale of ten, it would rank one with most people. It must be mixed into recipes to obscure its semi-fishy, seaweed-like taste.

At present spirulina is somewhat expensive, but prices will no doubt drop significantly if it becomes popular enough for demand to increase supply.

Storage

Lecithin should be refrigerated, especially in hot weather, since it contains fatty acids and, as always, rancidity is a threat. Fresh pollen must be refrigerated at all times and used within a period which should be stated on the label. Dried pollen, brewer's yeast, and spirulina require no special storage conditions.

Q. *I object to anything pertaining to the alcoholic beverage industry. Isn't brewer's yeast in that category?*

A. Back in the old days, when beer making was not dominated by chemicals, a by-product of brewing was a yeast which grew in the vats. This yeast was analyzed and revealed to be an excellent source of b-complex vitamins as well as some important trace minerals and proteins. This substance came to be known as brewer's yeast, although today's brewer's yeast has never seen the inside of a brewery. It is produced in laboratories, grown on molasses or whey, spray dried, and packed into drums for shipment to bulk dealers or packagers who put it into cans, bottles, or plastic bags. It is now more properly called *nutritional yeast*, the term "brewer's yeast" being primarily of historical interest.

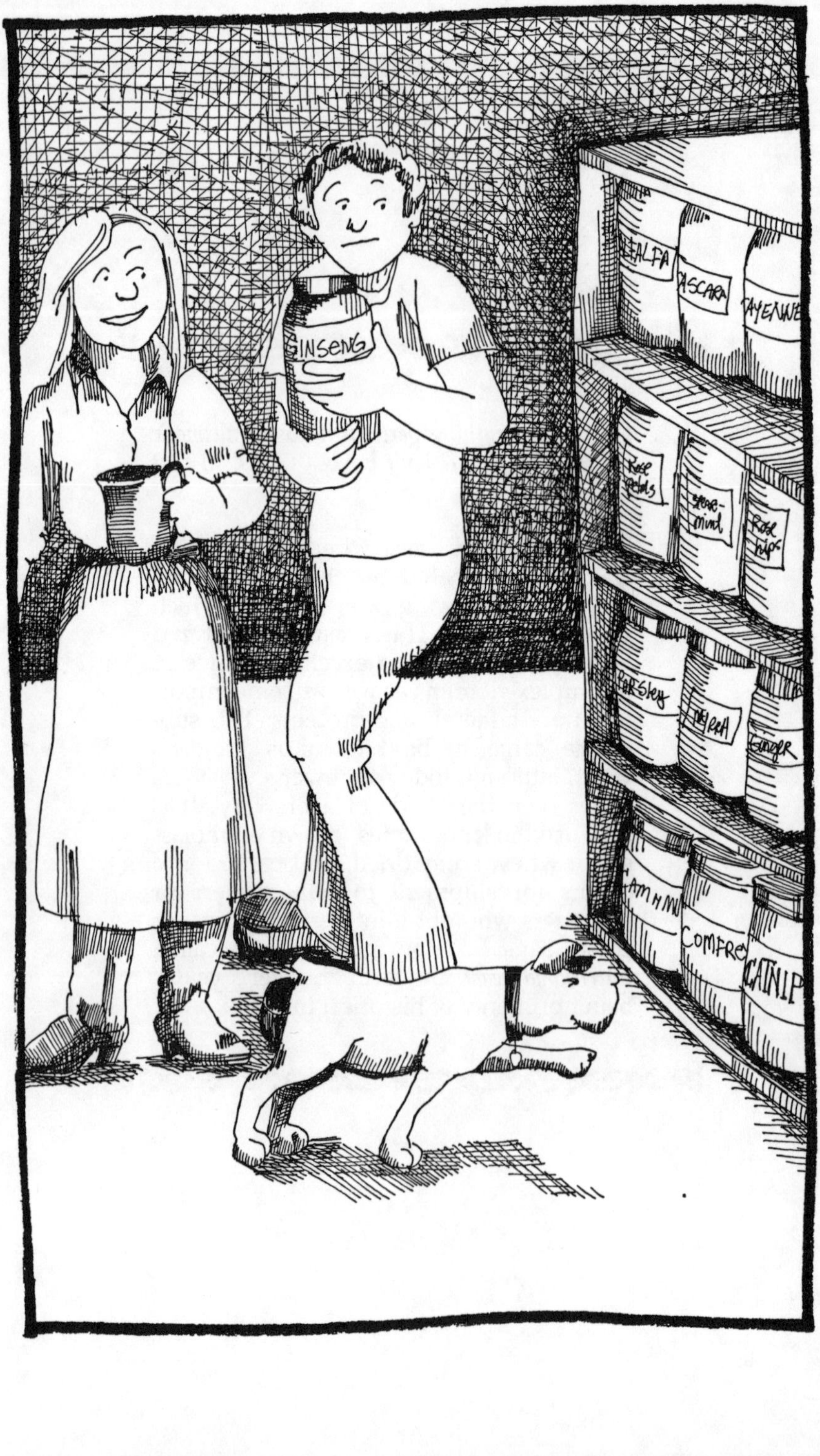
GINSENG
CASCARA
Rose petals
Rose hips
Parsley
MYRRH
Ginger
COMFREY
CATNIP

CHAPTER 19
Herbs, Spices, and Teas

Herbs

Although herbs have been used as folk medicines for thousands of years, it is only in the past five years or so that the general public has become aware of them. This is due in part to the growing interest in all things natural and the trend away from what is considered artificial or synthetic, and in part to an enormous marketing push by several major herb companies.

Historically, herbs have been used medicinally for everything from upset stomach to cancer. Sometimes they worked and sometimes they didn't. There is the temptation to consider them placebos, and their positive result psychosomatic, but in fact many herbs do contain substances which affect healing. A number of widely used drugs, such as digitalis, ephedrine, and reserpine, were derived from herbs, and I have no doubt that as more herbs are properly studied, more benefits will be discovered. However, some drugs derived from herbs are dangerous and thought to be carcinogenic.

In today's marketplace many people are reading the classical texts on herbal medicine, like Jethro Kloss's *Back to Eden* (Woodbridge Press edition, 1981, and others) and John Christopher's *School of Natural Healing* (Bi-World Publishers, 1976), and experimenting on their own with these traditional "cures." Herbs are used in a variety of ways: leaves and flowers are steeped in water as tea, called an *infusion;* roots and barks are boiled into a tea, called a *decoction;* concentrated in alcohol or vinegar, called a *tincture;* ground up and put into gelatin capsules; or made into various topical preparations like *poultices.*

It is far beyond our scope to do anything but touch upon the subject of herbs and their multitude of uses. There are literally thousands of active herbs and dozens of fine books describing their value, and I refer you to these should your curiosity be aroused. Be aware, though, that all herbs are not necessarily safe to use on a regular basis, as some contain toxic substances which may prove harmful if ingested often enough in sufficient amounts. As the Food and Drug Administration continues its investigation of herbs, we will see more and more of them pulled from shelves or labelled with appropriate warnings. When you go into an herb store or natural food store and start asking a lot of questions about what herbs are good for or what you can take for your arthritis, don't be put off if the clerk seems a little hesitant to give you any solid information. The law frowns on people who are not licensed physicians dispensing medical advice, and telling you that bats' wings and toads' tails will help your condition is considered prescribing medicine without a license. Many an herbalist has wound up in the slammer for just that.

Just so you don't feel totally cheated, the following is a list of just a dozen or so popular herbs and their traditional uses. Since Big Brother is undoubtedly watching, I am obligated to say here that this information is intended for educational purposes only and not to be prescriptive.

Alfalfa Leaves—high in minerals; good "spring tonic"
Catnip—settling to an upset stomach; will drive your cat up a wall
Cascara Sagrada—laxative
Cayenne—dilates blood vessels; breaks up mucous; very *hot*
Comfrey—soothing to irritated mucous membranes
Fennel—carminative (breaks up intestinal gas)
Ginger—causes sweating and brings on fever to break a cold
Goldenseal—antibiotic properties; tastes terrible
Lavendar—used in sachets and potpourris for great smell
Myrrh—rub on sore gums for relief
Parsley—diuretic; for quick water loss
Peppermint—aids digestion; breath freshener
Raspberry—helps prevent morning sickness in pregnancy
Rose Hips—high in vitamin C
Rose Petals—in sachets and potpourris
Spearmint—settling to the stomach

Any of these herbs may be brewed into a tea or taken in capsule form. To make a proper tea, bring water to a boil and take off the heat, add about a teaspoon of herb for each 8-ounce cup of water, and let it steep about fifteen or twenty minutes. This time period is critical since it takes that long for the alkaloids or active substances to be released into solution; otherwise the expected effects will be minimal.

Because lots of people don't have the time to brew up a tea, or simply don't like drinking teas, encapsulated herbs are becoming extremely popular. Practically every major herb and quite a few minor ones have been put into capsules and neatly packaged just like vitamin pills. Capsules are quite a bit more expensive but just as effective and very convenient. The latest rage is combinations of herbs based on traditional and modern formulations, each one tailored for some malady. These combinations are cleverly packaged and labelled to "suggest" that this one is good for asthma or that one for diabetes, but that connection is never actually stated on the label. Obviously, this is designed to keep the manufacturers safely inside the law.

Ginseng

An herb that deserves special attention is ginseng—definitely in a class by itself. It is a most unique plant, which has been the subject of more research than any other herb, with some very interesting findings. Most of this research has been done by Chinese, Korean, and Russian scientists, and the U.S. government has yet to accept the results as conclusive. As of this writing, the FDA still considers ginseng simply a beverage, and the only statement which may be made on the label is "used as a tea." Reported findings of experiments include (1) in elderly people, performance in physical tests increased significantly with ginseng use; (2) laboratory animals showed better reactions to stress, less fatigue; (3) ginseng destroyed 99 percent of one type of leukemia cells injected into mice; and (4) mice were able to swim longer when given ginseng.[1]

In general, scientists who have worked with ginseng consider it to be an "anti-stress" herb, in the sense that it appears to enable the user to better handle stress and stressful situations. Persons taking ginseng regularly report increased alertness and decreased fatigue. Apparently, however, like most beneficial substances, it can be overdone. Too much ginseng can result in hyperactivity symptoms and increased nervous activity. A cup of tea a day is possibly all that's necessary.

In natural food stores and elsewhere you will find ginseng marketed in a wide variety of ways: whole roots, powders, extracts, capsules, instant teas, and "gimmick" products like ginseng sodas, ginseng candies, and ginseng cosmetics. The whole unmolested root is the purest form, and it is by no means inexpensive. Ginseng, however, takes eight years to grow to maturity, and production requires exceptional skill and care, so prices are not wholly unjustified. Roots are "graded" by government agencies (theirs, not ours), and the higher the grade the greater the cost. People have been known to pay many thousands of dollars for a single root of extremely high quality, generally taken only once a year, but fairly good roots may be purchased in the $5 to $10 range. Roots come in white and red, the white being the natural root as it is grown and the red having been boiled along with other herbs, the identities of which are kept secret. Once you've obtained a satisfactory root, you may chew on a small piece if you like the taste, or brew it into a tea by simmering a slice in water for a few minutes and steeping for fifteen minutes more.

Ginseng powders also come in various grades, and a good quality powder may run about $5 an ounce. You may take this powder in capsule form by filling your own capsules or buying them ready made in bottles or bulk. Tea may be brewed from any ginseng powder by steeping one-half teaspoon in boiled water for fifteen to twenty minutes.

Ginseng extract is a thick dark brown, almost black, liquid with the consistency of honey. It comes in a small bottle and tea is made from it by mixing a tiny spoonful into hot water (the spoon comes with it).

Instant ginseng tea comes in little foil packages, and one of these dumped into hot water does the trick. These processed products are not usually of very good quality, however, and almost always contain dextrose as a sweetener.

That sham and scam exists in the marketing of ginseng products is not surprising. Anytime you have a semi-mysterious product surrounded by sweeping claims of near magical powers, the unscrupulous will not be far away if there's easy money to be made. Analytical tests were done on fifty-four products claiming to contain ginseng; 26 percent were found to have no ginseng whatsoever, and another 34 percent were so low in ginseng as to be considered insignificant. In all then, 60 percent of the tested products were judged to be "worthless" with respect to ginseng properties.[2] This is sad news, particularly for an industry that should be trying to regain public trust and vehemently avoiding the deceptive business practices so often found in the commercial marketplace.

Spices

Not all natural food stores carry extensive stocks of herbs, but almost all deal in spices, since they are such an integral part of natural food cooking. If you're lucky, your store dispenses spices in bulk. This is a most economical way to purchase them as long as you're willing to scoop them out and bag them up. When you buy spices in 1- and 2-ounce jars, you're often paying more for the jar than for the spice. We once ran a price comparison of spices sold in bulk in natural food stores to those in bottles at a number of supermarkets. The differences were phenomenal—often a spice selling at 35 cents an ounce in bulk was more than $8 for the same amount packaged in a nifty shaker bottle. And if your store does a brisk business in spices, chances are they will be much fresher.

If you really appreciate fresh spices, you might think about investing in a little grinder, manual or electric, and buying whole spices which you can grind as you need them.

Herb Tea

Any herb may be made into a tea, but the term "herb tea" usually refers to those which are drunk for pleasure only, rather than for their medicinal values. Many people begin trying herb teas in order to get away from coffee or ordinary black tea, which contains caffeine and tannic acid, both considered harmful. However, some herb teas do contain these substances, and if you wish to avoid them be wary of any blend containing black or green (matte) tea. Another advantage to herb tea is the presence of vitamins and minerals. Blends containing herbs like rose hips, lemon grass, alfalfa, and comfrey have significant amounts of important nutrients.

Herb teas may be sold in bulk or in tea bags. In either case, proper brewing is necessary to derive the full taste and benefit. Those accustomed to ordinary tea are used to letting their tea steep only a few minutes, just until it looks the right color. But herb tea should steep at least fifteen minutes for the best results. This time period serves the additional purpose of allowing the tea to cool down a bit—boiling hot liquids are not especially good for the system. If using bulk tea, one teaspoon to the cup is a good mix. You can just throw it in the pot and strain out the pieces after steeping or use one of the many brewing gadgets, like stainless steel tea-balls, teaspoons, tea scissors, or even reuseable cloth bags.

The most popular and widely marketed brand of herb tea is Celestial Seasonings. Many of their blends, like Red Zinger and Sleepytime have become household words in some areas of the country. Although most of their blends are for taste pleasure only, several have specific functions, which will only be alluded to on the labels, due to the usual legal restraints. Sleepytime, for example, contains certain herbs known to have relaxing or sedative effects, and thus is often used before bedtime. Morning Thunder is made up of green and black teas and is therefore high in caffeine for that morning pick-up.

Many stores dealing in bulk teas make up their own blends to compete with the popular brands or to simply broaden their selection. Usually, a laxative blend of some kind will be available. Laxative teas are reasonably safe for occasional use, but regular consumption is not recommended. If you're constipated often, you would do better to analyze your diet and root out the high fat, low fiber foods than to rely on laxatives, some of which, like senna leaves, may be rather irritating.

Coffee Substitutes

Herbs like chicory root and dandelion root are often used in blends with roasted barley to produce coffee substitutes. These are simply attempts to duplicate the taste of coffee without caffeine. They take a little getting used to but have helped many kick the caffeine habit. Pero, Pioneer, and Baroma are a few popular brands.

Selection and Storage

Herbs and herb teas should be sniffed and inspected for freshness. Although the shelf life is quite long, improper storage can affect the potency of herbs and spices. Most important is that they be kept tightly sealed and out of extended direct sunlight, as this will cause rapid deterioration.

Spices can get rancid or moldy, especially in hot, humid weather, and any long-term storage should be under refrigeration. Insects like weevils enjoy herbs and spices, and you can treat this condition just as you would with grains.

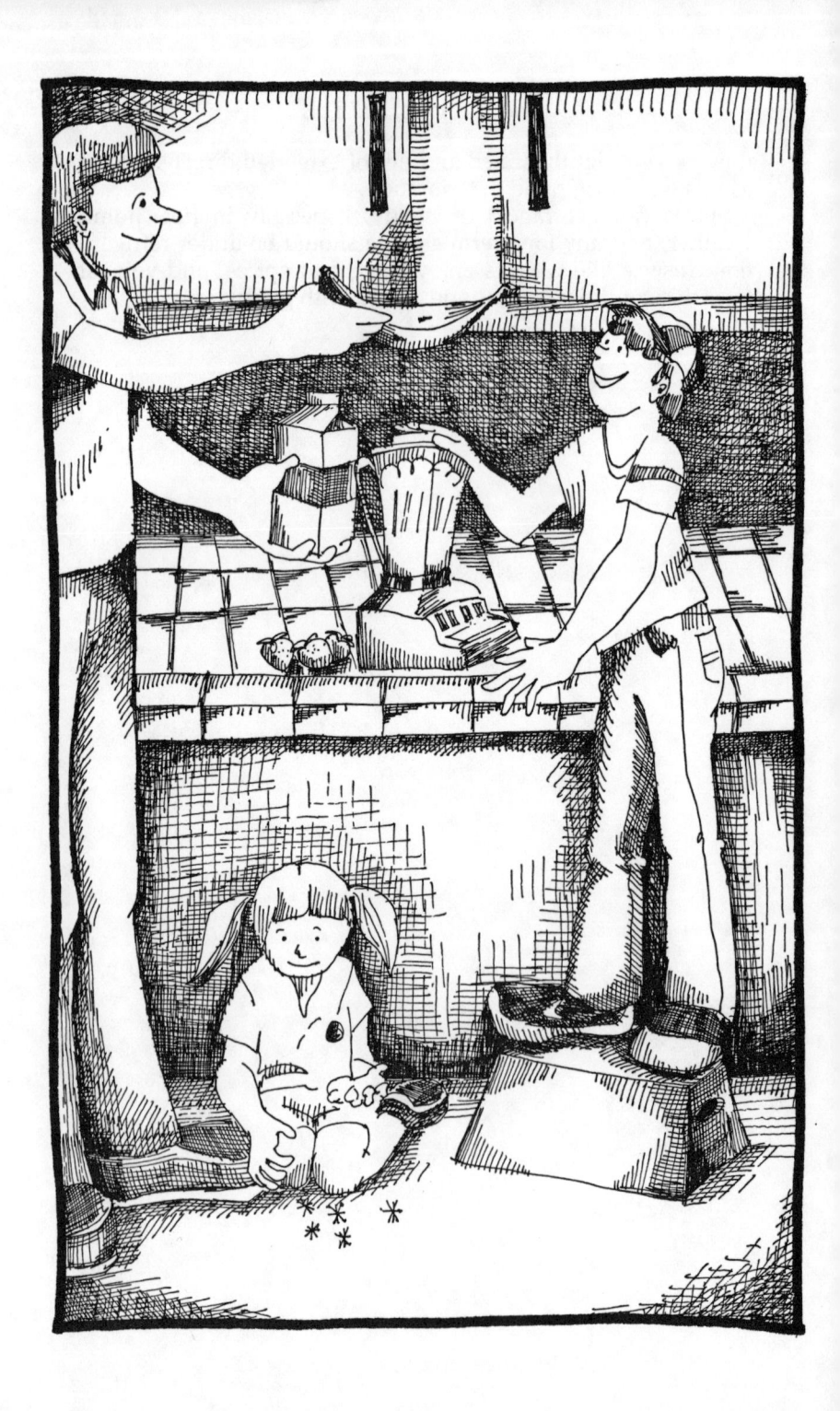

CHAPTER 20
Appliances

Although you may begin by picking up bags of trail mix for snacks and lunching on soyburgers and carrot juice at the local juice bar, sooner or later the natural foods experience will drive you into your own kitchen more and more often. This may be for economic reasons, but more likely because you want to have more personal control over the quality and preparation of your food. Though I do not deny that you could do quite well with no more than a sharp knife and a cast iron pot, our modern lifestyles and the need for variety in our diets often point us toward gadgets and appliances. A typical natural foods kitchen may contain a juicer, a blender, a flour mill, a nut and seed grinder, a yogurt maker, and perhaps even a water distiller or purifier. Let us look at just a few of these and see what choices are available and whether you really need them or not.

Juicers

If fruit and vegetable juices are an important part of your diet, you may be rightfully concerned over the purity and nutritional value of the juice you drink. As mentioned in Chapter 16, pasteurized juices have sustained certain losses of nutrients, and skepticism is warranted whenever purees and concentrates are used. The obvious way to eliminate these problems is by owning your own juicer and fully controlling the finished product. A juicer of your own, of course, also gives you the option of using organically grown fruits and vegetables if they are available to you.

A good juicer can produce juice from practically any fruit or vegetable, although you should be aware that coarse greens like parsley and spinach put a lot of wear and tear on your machine. And although you can certainly make orange juice, you will have to peel the oranges first, since the skin contains a bitter and potentially toxic oil.

Among the most popular brands of electrically operated juicers are the Acme, Champion, Norwalk, and Phoenix. Of these, the Acme is the best seller, but not necessarily the best. Although the Acme is a fine machine, it suffers, in my opinion, from two drawbacks. The first is that it does not continuously eject pulp and thus has to be stopped and emptied often as it fills up, and the second is that it really does little more than make juice. For roughly the same amount of money (both have a suggested retail of around $200) you can buy the *Champion*, which is pulp-ejecting and in addition to making juice will produce nut butters, purees, chopped ice, baby foods, and ice cream. For a low calorie, low fat ice cream substitute, try freezing peeled overripe bananas and running them through the *Champion*—tastes just like banana ice cream, with only one ingredient. This can be done with any fruit.

The Norwalk is a superior juicer by any standard, and it is capable of performing many functions. It is said to squeeze 30 percent more juice from fruits and vegetables, but one has to balance this gain against a $700 price tag. The Norwalk also involves a two-step juicing process, which many find a bit messy.

The Phoenix is a low cost ($90), recent European entry into the American market. It competes most directly with the Acme, to which it is similar.

If you're the type who resents energy-consuming appliances, you may prefer one of the inexpensive manual juicers. They do a good job if you don't mind the time and work involved. A manual juicer is simply a meat grinder with a special juice pressing attachment, and as such is a maintenance-free device with very few moving parts. With a few different cutter blades you can use it for grinding nuts, seeds, coffee, spices, or even meat.

Blenders

I'm not familiar enough with all the different brands of blenders on the market to be able to give you an intelligent consumer report, although I will say I've always found an Oster to be a sturdy, reliable machine. One thing I can say is this: Don't spend a lot of money on a blender just because it has 6000 different speeds all distinguished by cute little descriptions like "frappé" or "liquify." I mean, what is the difference between "mix" and "blend" anyway? Buy a blender with two speeds—high and low—that's all you'll ever need unless you just get your kicks from pressing buttons.

Blenders are useful for all sorts of food preparation involving puréeing and fine grinding, although we must admit that most of this could just as well be done with a wire whisk and a strong arm. One natural food treat, however, is inextricably bound to the blender—the smoothy. A smoothy is essentially a milk shake made with fruit and fruit juice instead of milk and ice cream. although some versions add these products as well. The basic smoothy, from which all others have evolved, consists of a banana and some apple juice. Usually these are blended together with a handful of ice cubes until a thick consistency is achieved, but I prefer the alternate method of freezing the banana first and then blending it with the juice. This eliminates the need for ice and produces a thicker, less watered down drink.

From this basic recipe you may let your imagination run rampant and create limitless concoctions. You can substitute other frozen fruits, like papaya or strawberries, for the banana, or put them in as additions. You certainly can use any juice you'd like or any combination of juices, and go on to build bigger and more complicated smoothies, adding nuts, dried fruits, ice cream, milk, yogurt, protein powder, wheat germ, bran, lecithin, bee pollen, yeast, carob powder, etc. Bear in mind that the more complex your smoothy becomes, the more likely it is to produce indigestion, so it's best to keep them reasonably simple. But then, it's your stomach.

Food Processors

Although nothing a food processor can do cannot be done with a blender and a sharp knife, people with large families and limited time may find a food processor worth the cost, particularly if your group is eating lots of chopped and grated vegetables. My experience has been that food processors are fun to play with for a while but after you've taken them apart, washed them, and put them back together a few times, you begin to wonder if you're really saving all that much time.

Mills

More and more people are choosing to bake their own whole grain breads for a number of reasons, including economy, guarantee of freshness, and control of ingredients. All of these are further strengthened if one mills one's own flour at home, rather than chancing the freshness of store bought.

Basically, you've got two decisions to make before purchasing a mill: manual or electric, and stone or steel. Electric mills offer the obvious convenience of dumping in a few pounds of grain, flicking a switch, and finding a few pounds of flour ready to go ten minutes later. Most will grind around twenty-five pounds per hour, but the hoppers have to be fed every four or five pounds, although you can rig up a hopper extension for grinding larger amounts. The disadvantages are the cost (starting around $250), and the tendency of all electrical gadgets to eventually break down and present you with repair bills. A good hand-operated mill will run you fifty bucks and will last a lifetime if not abused. Of course you can't flick a switch and walk away but it's good exercise. Some manual mills can be hooked up to a stationary bicycle so you can work off some calories while you prepare to eat some new ones.

Steel mills are cheaper than stone, but grind hot and so tend to destroy certain nutrients like vitamin E. Stone mills preserve these nutrients and also seem to be capable of finer adjustments. Remember, especially hard products like corn and beans should not be ground with stone, since they can cause excessive wear. A good idea might be to get the type of hand mill with convertible grinders, allowing you to use either steel or stone.

Water Purifiers and Distillers

If you're as skeptical about the safety of your local tap water as I am, you may be considering some sort of home system to provide you with clean water. Counter top or under the sink purifiers and distillers are becoming popular lately, and are available in a wide range of models and prices.

A purifier will remove bacteria and chemical pollutants as well as any large foreign particles, but will not remove heavy metals like lead or copper leached from your plumbing system. A distiller boils your tap water, producing steam which is then cooled in a coil and converted back into water, minus everything except hydrogen and oxygen and anything else that can be converted into a gas by boiling, like chlorine. To remove chlorine and any other unwanted gases, the final product may be run through activated charcoal, giving you 100% H_2O.

Distillers start at about $200, and purifiers are somewhat less; however, any good home handyman could build his own distiller rather easily. This could be made to run off an electrical heating element, a wood fire, or even by solar power.

Other Stuff

The natural food industry is not the least bit unaware of a universal infatuation with machines and gadgets, and there are no voids left to be filled. We will gladly sell you electric yogurt makers, cheese makers, and peanut butter machines; popcorn poppers, woks, and ice cream makers; mixers, dough-kneaders, and "total kitchen" machines that will do anything that would otherwise have to be done using simple tools, your two hands, and time. It is possible, however, delightfully possible, to have a totally nonelectric kitchen from which great meals can emerge—comforting to know as energy becomes more and more a luxury.

CHAPTER 21
Putting It All Together

Of Monkeys and Men

Although human beings are vastly superior to all other earthly creatures in the depth of their intellectual and spiritual capacities, physiologically we differ very little from our closest cousins, the apes. Our digestive systems, our glandular systems, and our skeletons and musculatures are much the same. I have no reason to believe our nutritional requirements are not also strikingly similar. Whether you believe we evolved from these creatures or were created as a distinct species does not alter our basic biological similarity. And in either case this animal body must be fed if it is to continue to house and transport our higher level functions. If we can admit to ourselves that our bodies need the same quality of nourishment as do those of our animal friends, then perhaps we ought to learn a little from them.

Animals do not process their foods. And except for the removal of inedible shells, husks, and peels, everything is eaten in its "as grown" state. Everything is also eaten raw, and in order to acquire enough calories animals must spend a great proportion of their day foraging for food and eating. This is an affordable luxury, of course, since animals have little else to do. I don't believe humans have been given their magnificent powers of creative reasoning to be wasted on the pursuit of sustenance. The intelligence of Man made two important discoveries which enabled him to nourish his body much more efficiently and free up some time so he could do things like invent the wheel and redecorate his cave. First, he discovered fire, which allowed him to take advantage of highly nutritious and plentiful foods like grain that were useless to him in the raw state. And second, he discovered the club, which, once mastered, showed him that animals are far more cooperative on the dinner table if they're dead. The principle was simple: let the animal spend his time finding food and processing it into protein and we can just whack him on the head and eat the finished product.

As Man developed further and social groups were formed, grain was cultivated and at last we could have some control over our food source. And although it would be neat to say that the discovery of weapons has not proved to be the biggest boon to mankind, without that club and its property of breaking necks Man would probably have not survived the Ice Age.

The point is this: we've used our brains in the past to deal with unusual circumstances—let's use them again. The Ice Age, with its accompanying scarcity of available plant food, threatened Man with extinction. The killing and eating of animals provided a creative alternative to that fate. Now, in spite of the fact that meat in those days was not polluted with chemicals, it still contained fats, cholesterol, and all the other negative properties and thus was only a slightly more healthful food than it is today. A wise man, however, does not become overly concerned about his cholesterol level when faced with extinction. Meat was the only game in town and it was rough times ahead for vegetarians.

But the Ice Age has passed, plant food is once again plentiful, and animal products have become increasingly unfit for those no longer concerned with survival of the species but with superior health. A new age is now upon us—the Processed Age—when the fundamental integrity of our natural food is being weakened not only by Man's technology but by his dependence upon animal foods. You see, the foods we obtain from animals, either by killing them, milking them, or pilfering their eggs, are processed foods. Perfectly good human foods like soybeans and grain are processed through animals to produce high protein, high fat, low fiber, nutritionally deficient products which are wreaking havoc with our health. The Ice Age didn't come overnight. It crept up slowly and steadily over thousands of years. Degenerative disease is creeping up on us just as methodically. In the U.S. today, one out of every four of us will get cancer and more than half of us will die from some form of hardening of the arteries. Is the Processed Age threatening us with an extinction of our own making?

Desirability of Common Foods Compared

Desirable		Less Desirable		Undesirable	
Unrefined Complex Carbohydrates	Unrefined Simple Carbohydrates	Refined Complex Carbohydrates	Refined Simple Carbohydrates	Protein/Fat Foods	100% Fat Foods
brown rice whole wheat whole barley millet buckwheat oats, corn, and all other whole grains whole grain cereals whole grain breads whole grain pasta potatoes, squash carrots, and all other vegies* all beans** (except soy and peanuts)	all fruits	white flour white rice white pasta bolted flours	white sugar brown sugar raw sugar honey molasses maple syrup other syrups	meat poultry fish milk cheese yogurt eggs soybeans*** peanuts*** nuts and seeds***	vegetable oil butter margarine lard

*Keep in mind that although most vegetables are predominantly carbohydrate they are too low in calories to form the basis of a sound diet. More concentrated sources of calories, such as grains, are needed to provide sufficient energy.
**Beans range above 20 percent protein and although useful in the diet for taste and variety, they should not be eaten too often.
***These are whole natural foods, and although high in fat may still be used in moderation in a sound diet.

How to Do It

If you have read this book carefully you should have a reasonably firm idea of what you ought and ought not to be eating. The next step is to put theory into practice. The diet I advocate has been eaten by primitive groups and peasants worldwide for all of recorded history, so its implementation doesn't require any special genius. What it does require is the grasping of two rather simple concepts. The first is understanding what natural foods are and how they may be identified. If you use the criteria outlined in Chapter 1 and observe the way in which they were applied to the various foods discussed throughout the book, you should have all the information necessary to make these judgments easily.

The second concept involves the different classes of foods and the degree to which they are emphasized in the overall diet. One way of classifying foods is according to the particular nutrient which is predominant in that food. We may then talk about unrefined complex carbohydrates, refined complex carbohydrates, unrefined simple carbohydrates, refined simple carbohydrates, protein/fat foods, and 100 percent fats. Naturally categories always overlap to some degree, but in general they remain distinct. Let us apply this system to some of the foods discussed in the chart on the opposite page.

As you can see, the most desirable foods are those consisting primarily of unrefined carbohydrates, particularly of the complex variety. Foods high in protein and fat are undesirable. This *does not mean* you don't need some protein and fat in your diet. You do, but you will get all you need by eating a variety of whole grains, fruits, and vegetables, without having to use any of the concentrated protein/fat foods listed on the right hand side of the chart. Fruits average 8 percent of calories as protein, potatoes and grains average 8 percent, and beans and green vegetables average 23 percent. Together, these foods average 13 percent protein, substantially more than your body needs (which is why you should keep your consumption of beans down to no more than three or four times a week).

Now, chances are you're not yet prepared to give up all animal foods forever, and would like to allow yourself small amounts from time to time. And considering how you've probably eaten most of your life, this is not unreasonable. The important point here is *emphasis*. In the typical Western diet the protein/fat food is the major focus of the meal. "Have some more chicken . . . have some more meat loaf . . . two eggs or three?" The carbohydrate representative is pushed off to the side, and usually consists of french fries drenched in oil, mashed potatoes whipped with butter and milk, white rice, white pasta, or white bread; and a four-inch bowl of head lettuce with tomato wedges is passed off as a salad, but only after three ounces of oil, vinegar, and sugar are dumped on it. It is a remarkable testimony to the resiliency of the human body that it can manage to endure such abuse for 70 years.

What I'm suggesting is that you change the emphasis of your meals so that the carbohydrate becomes the main focus. "Have some more brown rice . . . have some more corn . . . two baked potatoes or three?" That's what we want to hear. Shuffled off to the side you may have your small portion of rich food—meat, cheese, fish, etc.—something to spark up the meal if you need it. And by all means put something in that salad besides lettuce. If you use hearty tasting vegetables like grated carrots and beets, chopped bell peppers and green onions, mushrooms or radishes, you won't need globs of dressing to make it taste like something.

Thomas Jefferson used to say that he preferred to use only small amounts of meat "as a condiment." This makes excellent sense to me. If you require the taste of animal foods in your diet, use them as *tastes*, not as the central part of the meal. This is how Orientals traditionally eat. Rice and vegetables are the main course, with token amounts of fish, chicken, beef, or pork mixed in for flavor. Japanese who eat in this traditional manner suffer one-fifth the number of heart attacks Western peoples do. When Japanese move to Hawaii and adopt the typical Western high fat diet, their heart attack rate quickly equals ours.

Whether or not Man is eating himself into extinction remains to be seen. It is clear, however, that he is eating himself into a lot of trouble. Degenerative disease is on the rise wherever we look except in those places where people have clung to simple diets of whole foods. This descent into disease is not our inevitable fate, it is a fate of our own choosing, and we have the freedom and the right and the ability to alter it at any time. Don't hold your breath waiting for the government to tell you to stop eating animal foods and refined carbohydrates. The evidence against these foods exists, but it will be suppressed and obscured because there is too much money to be made by keeping it that way. You as an individual or as a family have to do it by yourself. Do it quietly or loudly, but do it.

Notes

Chapter 1

1. For a review of studies linking cholesterol levels to coronary heart disease, see Pritikin N: High carbohydrate diets: Maligned and misunderstood. *Journal of Applied Nutrition* 28:56–58, 1976. Also, see Shekelle RB, Shryock AM, Paul O, Lepper M, Stamler J., Liu S, and Raynor WJ: Diet, serum cholesterol, and death from coronary heart disease. *New England Journal of Medicine* 304:65, 1981, the results of a 20-year study involving 1900 middle-aged men showing that diet and cholesterol levels correlate with risk of coronary heart disease.
2. Hill MJ: Steroid nuclear dehydrogenation and colon cancer. *American Journal of Clinical Nutrition* 27:1475–1480, 1974.
   Wynder EL and Reddy BS: Metabolic epidemiology of colorectal cancer. *Cancer* 34:801–806, 1974.
3. Swank RA: *A Biochemical Basis of Multiple Sclerosis*, C. C. Thomas Publ., Springfield, IL, 1961.
4. Although it has been suggested that this same effect is achieved with polyunsaturated fat, a study by Blankenship clearly contradicts this notion. It was shown that an index of oxygen carrying capacity (2,3 DPG) was elevated when polyunsaturates replaced saturated fats in the diet despite no change in total fat (Blankenship J: personal communication).
5. Carroll KK: Experimental evidence of dietary factors and hormone-dependent cancers. *Cancer Research* 35:3374–3383, 1975.
   Carroll KK and Hopkins GJ: Dietary polyunsaturated fat versus saturated fat in relation to mammary carcinogenesis. *Lipids* 14:155–158, 1978.
   Nishizuka Y: Biological influence of fat intake on mammary cancer and mammary tissue: Experimental correlates. *Preventative Medicine* 7:218–224, 1978.
6. Ernst E and Levy RI: Diet, hyperlipidemia and atherosclerosis. In Goodhart RS and Shils ME: *Modern Nutrition in Health and Disease*, 6th ed., Lea and Febiger, Philadelphia, 1980, p. 1047.
7. See note no. 1.
8. In some age groups there is not a good correlation between total serum cholesterol and heart attack risk. However, it is becoming increasingly clear that more important than the total cholesterol is the ratio between two types of cholesterol: low density lipoproteins (LDL) and high density lipoproteins (HDL). HDL's are large molecules which appear to be beneficial to the system, acting perhaps as "sweepers" to clean up the arteries, while LDL's seem to be the problem ones. When this relationship was looked at carefully, it was clear that risk of coronary heart disease was positively correlated with LDL levels in all age groups. (Stamler J: Population Studies. In Levi RI et al: *Nutrition, Lipids and Coronary Heart Disease*, Raven Press, New York, 1979, p. 59.
9. Ten percent would meet the recommendations of the Food and Nutrition Board and this is admittedly in excess of what is actually needed. Generally these recommended percentages are double the minimum needs, to allow for a "margin of safety."

Notes

10. Evans N and Risley EH: High protein ration as a cause of nephritis. *California and Western Medicine* 23: no. 4: 437–442, 1925.
    Schilling E: *Nutrition Abstracts and Reviews* 33:114, 1963.
11. Walker RM and Linkswiler HM: Calcium retention in the adult human male as affected by protein intake. *Journal of Nutrition* 102:1297, 1972.
    Wachman A and Bernstein DS: Diet and osteoporosis. *Lancet* 1:958–959, 1968.
    Mazess RB and Mather W: Bone mineral content of North Alaskan Eskimos. *American Journal of Clinical Nutrition* 27:916–925, 1974.
12. Margen S, Chu JY, Kaufman NA, Calloway DH: Studies in calcium metabolism. I. The calciuretic effect of dietary protein. *American Journal of Clinical Nutrition* 27:584–589, 1974.
13. Costill DL: The drinking runner. In Higdon H: *The Complete Diet Guide for Runners and Other Athletes*, World Publ., Mountain View, CA, 1978, pp. 155–156.
14. For an extensive discussion of fiber and its relationship to disease and constipation, see Burkitt D: *Eat Right—To Stay Healthy and Enjoy Life More*. Arco, New York, 1979.
15. Ershoff BH: Protective effects of cholestyramine in rats fed a low-fiber diet containing toxic doses of sodium cyclamate or amaranth (39373). *Proceedings of the Society of Experimental Biology and Medicine* 152:253–256, 1976.
16. Alliteration, thanks to Nathan Pritikin.
17. Flynn, et al: *Irish Journal of Medical Science* 146:285, 1977.
18. Donald P, Pitts GC and Pohl SL: Body weight and composition in laboratory rats: Effects of diets with high or low protein concentration. *Science* 211:185–186, 1981.
19. Lemon FR and Kuzma JW: A biologic cost of smoking. *Archives of Environmental Health* 18:950–955, 1969.
    Phillips, RL, Lemon FR, and Hammond C: Coronary heart disease mortality among Seventh-day Adventists with differing dietary habits. *Abstract American Public Health Association meeting*, Chicago, IL, November 16–20, 1975.
20. Krick EH: Why some people seem immune to cancer. *Life and Health*, Cancer Prevention Special, pp. 12–14.
21. Belloc NB and Breslow L: Relationship of physical health status and health practices. *Preventative Medicine* 1:409–421, 1972.
    Belloc, NB: Relationship of health practices and mortality. *Preventative Medicine* 2:67–81, 1973.
    Breslow L: A quantitative approach to the World Health Organization definition of health. *International Journal of Epidemiology* 1: no. 4: 347–355, 1972.
    Breslow L: Reducing risk factors. *Preventative Medicine* 7:449–458, 1978.

Chapter 3

1. Sanchez A, Reeser HL, Lau HS, Yahiku PY, Willard RE, McMillan PJ, Cho SY, Magie AR and Register UD: Role of sugars in human neutrophilic phagocytosis. *American Journal of Clinical Nutrition* 26:1180–1184, 1973.

Chapter 4

1. Nasset ES: Role of the digestive tract in the utilization of protein and amino acids. *Journal of the American Medical Association* 164:172–177, 1957.
    Yang SP, Clark HE, and Vail GE: Effects of varied levels and a single daily supplement of lysine on the nutritional improvement of wheat flour proteins. *Journal of Nutrition* 75:241–246, 1961.

2. Even in situations where unfortunate people are claimed to be suffering from protein-deficiency diseases like kwashiorkor and marasmus, the real problem is caloric deficiency. In other words, the lack of sufficient protein is due to the lack of sufficient calories. Once the individuals get enough calories, they have enough protein. Whenever discussions of calorie-protein deficiencies take place, it seems that we soon forget about the calories and confine the discussion to protein. It is possible to find individuals receiving enough calories but still deficient in protein, but this is rare and requires a rather obviously limited diet.

Viteri FE and Arroyave G: Protein-calorie malnutrition. In Goodhart RS and Shils ME: *Modern Nutrition in Health and Disease*, Lea and Febiger, Philadelphia, 1973, p. 607.

Hegsted DM: Deprivation syndrome or protein-calorie malnutrition. *Nutrition Reviews* 30:51–54, 1972.

3. Wynder EL: The dietary environment and cancer. *Journal of the American Dietetic Association* 71:385–391, 1977.

Narisawa T, Magadia NE, Weisburger JH and Wynder EL: Promoting effect of bile acids on colon carcinogenesis after intrarectal installation of N-Methyl-N'-nitro-N-nitrosoquanidine in rats. *Journal of the National Cancer Institute* 53:1093–1095, 1974.

Reddy, BS, Narisawa T, Weisburger JH, and Wynder EL: Brief communication: Promoting effect of sodium deoxycholate on colon adenocarcinomas in germ free rats. *Journal of the National Cancer Institute* 56:441–442, 1976.

Hill MJ, Draser BS, Aries V, Crowther JS, Hawksworth G, Williams REO: Bacteria and etiology of cancer of large bowel. *Lancet* 1:95–103, 1971.

4. For a good review of the literature concerning saturated fat and these diseases see Scharffenberg, JA: *Problems With Meat*, Woodbridge Press, Santa Barbara, 1979.

5. Enos WF, Beyer JC, and Holmes RH. Pathogenesis of coronary disease in American soldiers killed in Korea. *Journal of the American Medical Association* 158:912–915, 1955.

Also, the same type of result was shown during the Vietnam War (McNamara JJ, Molot MA, Stremple JF, and Cutting RT: Coronary artery disease in combat casualties in Vietnam. *Journal of the American Medical Association* 216:1185–1187, 1971.

6. See note no. 5.

7. Grace JT, Mirand EA, and Mount DT: Relationship of viruses to malignant disease. *American Medical Association Archives of Internal Medicine* 105:482–490, 1960.

Shimkin ME: *Ca—A Cancer Journal for Clinicians* 24: no. 3: 189, 1974.

8. Chenarin I: *The Megaloblastic Anaemias*, Oxford, Blackwell Scientific Publ, 1969, pp. 708–714.

9. *Nutrition Reviews* 38:274–275, 1980.

Chapter 5

1. Lately there is growing opinion that some saturated fatty acids may not be harmful, at least with respect to elevating blood cholesterol levels. Saturated fatty acids differ in numbers of carbons in the chain. Stearic has 18, palmitic 16, myristic 14, and lauric 12. Shorter-chain fatty acids are metabolized differently and do not tend to elevate blood cholesterol levels. Of the longer-chain fatty acids, myristic and lauric are not found in large quantities in the foods we commonly eat, the exception being coconut, which has as high as 40 percent lauric acid and thus tends to elevate cholesterol. The two most

commonly found in our foods in large amounts are stearic and palmitic fatty acids. Recent evidence demonstrates that stearic acid may not be a problem in the cholesterol story at all, but palmitic is. Foods that contain a lot of palmitic acid from the most to the least are palm kernel oil, animal foods of all types, chocolate, cottonseed oil, and avocado.

2. Keys A: Cardiology: The essentiality of prevention. *Minnesota Medicine* August 1969, 1191–1196.
3. Press M, Hartop PJ, and Prottey C: Correction of essential fatty acid deficiency in man by the cutaneous application of sunflower seed oil. *Lancet* 1:597, 1974.
4. Tanaka N and Portman OW: Effects of diet and chenodeoxycholic acid on cholesterol gallstones, plasma, and biliary lipids in squirrel monkeys. *Circulation Supplement III* 271, 1974.
5. See note no. 5, Chapter 1.
6. National Economics Division, Economics, Statistics and Cooperative Service, U.S. Dept. of Agriculture: Fats and Oils Situation, July 1980, Washington, D.C., p. 22.
7. Armstrong ML, Warren ED, and Connor WE: Regression of coronary atheromatosis in rhesus monkeys. *Circulation Research* 27:59–67, 1970.
Wissler RW and Vesselinovitch D: Studies of regression of advanced atherosclerosis in experimental animals and man. *Annals of the New York Academy of Science* 275:363–376, 1976.
8. Broitman SA, Vitale JJ, Vavrousek-Jakuba E, and Gottlieb LS: Polyunsaturated fat, cholesterol, and large bowel tumorigenesis. *Cancer* 40:2455–2463, 1977.
Pearce ML and Dayton S: Incidence of cancer in men on a diet high in polyunsaturated fat. *Lancet* 1:464–467, 1971.

Chapter 6

1. Matsudo H, Hodgkin NM, and Tanaka A: Japanese gastric cancer: Potentially carcinogenic silicates (talc) from rice. *Archives of Pathology* 97:366–368, 1974.
2. Stemmerman GN and Kolonel LN: Talc-coated rice as a risk factor for stomach cancer. *American Journal of Clinical Nutrition* 31:2017–2019, 1978.
3. Munoz JM: High fiber diets may lower serum cholesterol levels. *Research News*, U.S. Dept. of Agriculture, April 13, 1978.

Chapter 7

1. *Nutrition Reviews* 38:159–160, 1980.
Trowell H: Ischemic heart disease and dietary fiber. *American Journal of Clinical Nutrition* 25:926–932, 1972.
Trowell H: Fiber: A natural hypocholesteremic agent. *American Journal of Clinical Nutrition* 25:464–465, 1972.
2. Rackis JJ: in Smith AK and Circle SJ (eds): *Soybeans: Chemistry and Technology*, vol. 1, AVI Pub. Co., Westport, CT, 1978, pp. 158–202.

Chapter 8

1. Halsted JA *et al:* A conspectus of research on zinc requirements of man. In Irwin MI: *Nutritional Requirements of Man*, The Nutrition Foundation, Washington, D.C., p. 223.
Mason KE: A conspectus of research on copper metabolism and requirements of man. *Ibid*, p. 502.

1. Bowering J and Sanchez AM: A conspectus of research on iron requirements of man. *Ibid*, p. 327.
2. Kritchevsky D: Fiber, lipids, and atherosclerosis. *American Journal of Clinical Nutrition* 31:S65–S72, 1978.
   Kay RN and Truswell AS: Effects of citrus pectin on blood lipids and fecal steroid excretion in man. *American Journal of Clinical Nutrition* 30:171–175, 1977.
   van Berge-Henegouwen GP, Huybregts AW, van de Werf S, Demacker P, and Schade RW: Effect of a standardized wheat bran preparation on serum lipids in young healthy males. *American Journal of Clinical Nutrition* 32:794–798, 1979.

Chapter 10

1. Hundley JM: Influence of fructose and other carbohydrates on niacin requirement of rat. *Journal of Biological Chemistry* 181:1–9, 1949.
   Piering WF, Lemann J, and Lennon EJ: The effect of carbohydrate administration on urinary calcium and magnesium excretion. *Clinical Research* 16:393, 1968.
   Lindeman RD, Adler S, Yiengst MJ, and Beard ES: Influence of various nutrients on urinary divalent cation excretion. *Journal of Laboratory and Clinical Medicine* 70:236–245, 1967.
   Lennon EJ, Piering WF, and Lemann J: A Possible mechanism for diminished renal tubular calcium and magnesium reabsorption after glucose ingestion. *Clinical Research* 16:388, 1968.

Chapter 14

1. Enright JB: Thermal inactivation of Coxiella burnetti and its relation to pasteurization of milk. *U.S. Public Health Monograph* 47, 1957.
2. Shimkin ME: *Ca—A Cancer Journal for Clinicians* 24: no. 3: 189, 1974.
3. Wales A: The role of the combination of sucrose and milk in diabetes milletus. *American Journal of Clinical Nutrition* 29:689–690, 1976.
   Wales A: The role of the combination of sucrose and milk in diabetes milletus. *American Journal of Clinical Nutrition* 31:559–560, 1978.

Chapter 15

1. Akizuki S: *Physical Constitution and Food*, Nagazaki, 1965, p. 238.
   Heritage F: *Composition and Facts About Foods*, Health Research, Mokelumne, CA, 1968, p. 36.

Chapter 18

1. This of course is far too high a percentage of protein if spirulina is used as a significant contributor to caloric intake. However, this becomes academic if it is used only as a supplement, one tablespoon supplying only 6 grams of protein.

Chapter 19

1. Kronick J: *Whole Foods* 1: no. 11, 30, 1978.
2. Ziglar W: *Whole Foods* 2: no. 4, 28, 1978.

Index

aduki beans (*see* azuki beans)
aflatoxin, 185
agar-agar, 233
alcohol, 27
Alfalfa Dip (recipe), 209
All-Grain Mush (recipe), 129
almonds, 178–179
amino acids, 54
appendicitis, 29
Apple Crisp (recipe), 171
apricot kernel oil, 76
arame, 233
artery closure, and saturated fat, 68–69
asbestos, in white rice, 92
atherosclerosis, 32, 59
avocado, and cholesterol levels, 24
avocado oil, 76
azuki beans, 104

baked goods, packaged, 147–150
baking powder, 143–144
baking soda, 143
banana chips, 200
Banana Cream Pie (recipe), 171
barley
  scotch, 89
  whole, 89
Barley-Mushroom Casserole (recipe), 102–103
Beanburgers (recipe), 251
beans, 105–114 (*see also* specific types)
  and flatulence, 105–106
  preparation, 112
  selection and storage, 111–112
  value as food, 106
bee pollen, 258–260
  storage, 260

Bible Bread, 149
black beans, 106
Black Beans and Rice (recipe), 113
blackeyed peas, 106–107
blackstrap molasses, 161
blanching, of nuts, 109
blended oils, 75–76
blenders, 272–273
bran, 119–120, 144
  and constipation, 119–120
  and loss of minerals, 119–120
  rice, 119
Bran Muffins (recipe), 155
Brazil nuts, 179–180
breatharian, 47
brewer's yeast, 257–258
  storage, 260
brown sugar, 159
buckwheat, 89
bulgur, 120
butter, 216

calcium, in chicken, 282
caloric density, 34–37
camp mixes, 191
cancer
  colon, 23
  colon, and fiber, 29
  and polyunsaturated oils, 24, 79
candy bars, 200–201
carbohydrates
  complex, 30–31
  refined, 26–28, 30
  simple, 30
carob flour, 140
carob powder, 140
carob-coated snacks, 199
carrot juice, 240–241
cashews, 180–181

catsup, 232
cereals
  breakfast, 117–129
  cream, 118
  hulled whole, 117
  popular, and sugar, 123–124
  preparation, 128
  puffed, 118–119
  selection and storage, 127
  shredded, 118
chapatti, 149
cheese, 214–216
  low fat, 215
  natural, 214
  rennetless, 215
cheese food, 214–215
chemicals, in food, 31–32
chestnuts, 181
chia seeds, 207–208
chickpeas, 107
Chili (recipe), 80
chips, 152–153
cholesterol
  blood levels, 23–25
  blood levels, and beans, 106
  blood levels, and fiber, 29
  in foods, 24–25
coconut, 181
  in baking, 144–145
coconut oil, 75
coffee substitutes, 268
cola drinks, 241–242
colonic irrigation, 50–51
constipation, 29–30
  and bran, 119–120
cookies and cakes, 150–152
cooking, and nutrients, 47–48
corn, 90
corn flour, 138
corn germ, 123
corn oil, 73
cornmeal, 138–139
coronary artery disease, 23
  and fiber, 29
cottonseed oil, 75
cowpeas, 106–107
crackers, 152
cress seeds, 207

dairy (and egg) substitutes, 222–225
dairy products, desirability in diet, 221–222

dal (*see* dhal)
date sugar, 160
dates, 189
dhal, 107
diabetes, 29
diastatic malt, 161
diet
  high protein, 36
  ideal, 62–64
diverticulitis, 29
dried fruit, 187–190
  desirability in diet, 176–177
  drying process, 188
  selection and storage, 190
  sulfured, 188
dulse, 233

eggs, 220–222
  brown, 221
  fertile, 220
  raw, 221
egg replacers, 226
enrichment, of white flour, 87- 88, 134–135
enzymes, plant, 47–48, 204
exercise, and diet, 284–285

fasting, 49–50
fat, 23–24, 67–69, 83–84
  composition in foods (tables), 83–84
  monounsaturated, 23–24, 68–69
  polyunsaturated, 23–24, 68–69
  saturated, 23–24, 67–69
fatty acids, 67–69
fava beans, 111
fiber, 29–30
  as protection against toxins, 33
figs, dried, 189
filberts, 181–182
fish, as a protein source, 59–61
flakes, 118
flax seeds, 207–208
flaxseed oil, 76
flour, 131–142
  organic, 141
  selection and storage, 141–142
  whole wheat (*see* whole wheat flour)
food combining, 49
food processors, 273
French Apple Tart (recipe), 172
fructose, 159–160

Index

fruit, dried (see dried fruit)
fruit butters, 192
fruit juice, 137–240
   concentrates, 239
   raw vs. pasteurized, 238
fruitarian, 47

Gado Gado (recipe), 193
gallstones, 29
garbanzo beans, 107
ginseng, 265–267
glucose, 157–158
gluten, in wheat, 94
gluten flour, 139–140
Gourmet Rice (recipe), 103
gout, 26
grains, 87–103 (see also specific types)
   and insect infestation, 96–97
   moldy, 95
   organic, 100–101
   preparation, 101–103
   selection and storage, 95–96
granola, 125–127
great northern beans, 111
grits, 117, 120

Hazel nuts, 181–182
hemorrhoids, 29
herb tea, 267–268
herbs, 263–269
   storage, 268–269
hiatus hernia, 29
high blood pressure, and salt, 28
hijiki, 233
hominy grits, 120
honey, 163–166
   comb, 165
Hummous (recipe), 113
hydrogenated fat, 69–70
hydrogenation, 69–70

ice cream
   desirability in diet, 218–219
   natural, 219
insects, in natural foods, 96–97
Italian Buckwheat Rolls (recipe), 103
Italian Nonmeat Balls (recipe), 252

juice
   desirability in diet, 241

   fruit (see fruit juice)
   vegetable (see vegetable juice)
juicers, 271–272

kefir, 218
kefir cheese, 218
kelp, 145
kidney beans, 107
kidneys, and excess protein, 25–26
kombu, 233

leavening, 142–144
lecithin, 255–257
   storage, 260
legumes, 105
lentils, 107–108
linoleic acid, 67–68, 78–79
longevity, and diet, 38

macadamia nuts, 182
macrobiotics, 46–47
malt syrup, 161
maple syrup, 161–163
margarine, 222–223
mayonnaise, 229–230
meat analogs (and substitutes), 248–249
meat eating, 56–57
meats
   without additives 247–248
   without additives; storage, 251
Middle East Vegetable Stew (recipe), 81
milk
   acidophilus, 213
   and calcium needs, 58
   cow's, compared to human milk, 57–59
   goat's, 213–214
   powdered, 145
   raw certified, 211–213
   synthetic nutrients in, 213
Miller's bran (see bran)
millet, 90
   as cereal, 120–121
mills, grain, 274
miso, 232–233
molasses, 160–161
mucousless diet, 48
muesli, 121
mung beans, 108

muscillagenous seeds, 207–208
mush, 121
Mushroom Gravy (recipe), 80

natural food
  definition, 19–20
  economics, 37–38
navy beans, 111
nectar, 240
nigari, 224
nitrogen flushing
  of oils, 77
  of wheat germ, 123
nori, 233
nut butters, 191–192
nut milk, 225
Nut and Seed Loaf (recipe), 192–193
nutritional yeast, 257–258
nuts, 177–185 (*see also* specific types)
  chopped, 178
  (and seeds) desirability in diet, 175–176
  raw vs. roasted, 178
  selection and storage, 184–185
  shelled vs. unshelled, 177–178

oatmeal, 121
oats, 90
  rolled, 121
  steel cut, 122
obesity, 33–37
oils, 67–82 (*see also* specific types)
  in bulk, 77
  and cancer, 77
  cold pressed, 71
  desirability in diet, 77–79
  expeller pressed, 70
  and gallstones, 77
  manufacture of, 70
  nitrogen flushed, 77
  oxidation of, 72–73
  rancidity in, 72–73
  storage, 72–73, 76–77
  unbleached, 72
  unrefined, 71–72
olive oil, 74–75
organic foods, 97–101
osteoporosis, 26

palm kernel oil, 75

papaya, dried, 189
pasta
  refined, 153
  whole grain, 153–154
pasteurization, of milk, 212
pastry flour, whole wheat, 138
Peanut, Tofu, and Sesame Soup (recipe), 193–194
peanut butter, 191–192
peanut oil, 74
peanuts, 108–109
Peanuts and Bulgur (recipe), 114
peas
  split, 109–110
  whole, 109
pecans, 182–183
pepitas, 186
pesticides, 99
pignolias, 183
pine nuts, 183
pineapple, dried, 189
pink beans, 111
pinto beans, 110
pistachio nuts, 183
pita bread, 149
popcorn, 90–91
porridge, 121
Potato Chips, No Oil (recipe), 82
pregnancy, and protein, 282–283
preservatives, 31–32
preserves, 192
protein, 25–26, 53–64
  and body building, 56
  in children, 282
  complementing, 48, 54–55
  needs, 55–56
pulses, 105
pumpkin seeds, 186

raisins, 189
rapeseed oil, 76
Ratatouille (recipe), 81
raw foodist, 47–48
raw milk, 211–213
raw sugar, 159
red beans, 111
Refried Beans (recipe), 114
rice
  brown, 91
  brown, vs. white rice, 87–88
  mochi, 91–92

Index

sweet, 91–92
  white, 92
  white, and asbestos, 92
rice polish, 122
rice syrup, 161
Russian Dressing (recipe), 234
rye, 93
  flour, 138

safflower oil, 73–74
  cooking with, 74
salad dressings, 230
salt, 28–29
sea salt, 146
sea vegetables, 233
seasonings
  dry, 230–231
  liquid, 231
seaweed, 233
seed butters, 192
seed cheese, 225
seeds, 185–187 (*see also* specific types)
  selection and storage, 187
semolina flour, 93
sesame oil, 74
sesame seeds, 186–187
shoyu, 231
Sloppy Joes (recipe), 252
snacks
  desirability in diet, 197–198
  storage, 201
soda pop, 241–242
sodium, 28–29
soft drinks, 241–242
sorghum, 93
sorghum syrup, 161
soups, packaged, 232
sourdough, 143
Soy Butter (recipe), 226
soy flour, 139
soy oil (soya oil, soybean oil), 73
soy sauce, 231
soybeans (soya beans), 110–111
  toxins in, 111
soymilk, 224
  compared to cow's milk, 224
spices, 267
  storage, 269
spirulina, 260
Split Pea Chowder (recipe), 113

sproutarian, 47
Sprout Bread (recipe), 209
sproutbread, 150
sprouting, 205–208
sprouting buckwheat, 208
sprouting guide, 209
sprouts
  economics, 205
  nutritional value, 203–205
stone grinding, of flour, 137–138
sucrose, 157
sugar, raw (*see* raw sugar)
sugar, white, 157–158
sulfur dioxide, in dried fruits, 188
Sun Dip (recipe), 194
sunflower oil, 74
sunflower seeds, 187
Sweet and Sour Lentil Soup (recipe), 114
sweet tooth, 167–170
sweeteners
  desirability in diet, 166–167 (*see also* specific types)

Tabouli (recipe), 128
tamari, 231
tempeh, 250
textured vegetable protein (T.V.P.), 248–249, 250–251
  storage, 251
tofu, 223–224, 250
  storage, 251
tortillas, 149
toxins, and fasting, 49–50
trail mixes, 191
triticale, 93
turbinado sugar (*see* raw sugar)
turtle beans, 106
T.V.P. (*see* textured vegetable protein)

unbleached white flour, 139
uric acid, 26

vanilla, 146–147
varicose veins, 29
vegan, 46–47
vegetable juice, 240–241
vegetarian
  lacto-, 46
  lacto-ovo-, 45–46
  strict, 46

Vegie-Nut Stir Fry (recipe), 193
Vegie Salad Dressing (recipe), 234
vinegar, 230
vitamin B12, 61
　in miso, 232
vitamin E, in wheat germ oil, 76
vitamin requirements, 26–27

wakame, 233
walnut oil, 76
walnuts, 184
water
　bottled, 242–243
　carbonated, 244–245
　distilled, 244
　mineral, 244
　tap, 242–243
water distillers (and purifiers), 274–275
weevils, 96–97
weight loss, and complex carbohydrates, 35–36
wheat
　berries, 94
　cracked, 120
　durum, 93
　hard, 94
　pastry, 94
　soft, 94
　spring, 94
　winter, 94
wheat germ, 122–123
wheat germ oil, 76
wheatgrass, 204–205
white beans, 111
white flour
　enriched, 134–135
　production of, 132–133
white sugar (*see* sugar, white)
Whole Wheat Bread, Basic (recipe), 154–155
whole wheat flour, 135–138
　fresh-ground, 136–137
　pastry, 138
　vs. enriched white flour, 134–135
　vs. white flour, 133
winged beans, 111
yeast, baking, 142–143
yeast, brewer's (*see* brewer's yeast)
Yeast Cheese (recipe), 226
yeast, nutritional (*see* nutritional yeast)
yellow-D sugar (*see* brown sugar)
yogurt, 216–218
　making your own, 217–218
yogurt-coated snacks, 200